NUTRITION AND DIET RESEARCH PROGRESS

FOCUS ON NUTRITION IN CHILD-JUVENILE POPULATIONS IN A MEDITERRANEAN AREA

NUTRITION AND DIET RESEARCH PROGRESS

Additional books in this series can be found on Nova's website under the Series tab.

Additional e-books in this series can be found on Nova's website under the e-book tab.

FOCUS ON NUTRITION IN CHILD-JUVENILE POPULATIONS IN A MEDITERRANEAN AREA

TEODORO DURÁ-TRAVÉ
EDITOR

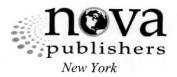

nova
publishers
New York

Library of Congress Cataloging-in-Publication Data

ISBN: 978-1-63463-223-2

Library of Congress Control Number: 2014952256

Published by Nova Science Publishers, Inc. † New York

CONTENTS

PREFACE

Food and eating patterns are important cultural and social referents of the different societies. During the past years, dietary habits have been considered social and sanitary indicators of a particular population due to scientific studies related to diet and health condition. The idea of "Mediterranean diet" comes from the eating habits that are traditional part of the culture of certain countries of the Mediterranean area. The fact that every food group, in appropriate proportions, is included in the Mediterranean diet has aroused great nutritional interest, being its main focus the balance calorie and nutrient intake through the combination of fruits and vegetables, pasta and rice, legumes, dairy products, fish and red meat and olive oil as cooking fat.

In addition to this recognition of the Mediterranean diet as a prototype of varied and nutritional diet, it has been observed that it contributes to prevent cardiovascular diseases, hypertension, diabetes, cancer, etc. and, overall, to a higher life expectancy.

However, it is outstanding the series of changes that society is going through nowadays and it affects as well the feeding habits of the population through the industrialization of the food chain or the mass production of processed food. The acceptance of a dietary pattern that allows an excessive intake of food from animal origin, specially meat and derivatives, and added sugars has meant a detriment of the intake of cereals, vegetables and fruits leading to an increase of saturated fat and cholesterol in diet.

This damage of dietary patterns in society has begun a fear of the disappearance of Mediterranean diet. This fear highly justifies the study of the quality of feeding habits in general population and the focus on the most sensitive sectors such as children and youth.

The aim of this book is to evaluate the dietary pattern of a young population which includes children and undergraduates from a Mediterranean area, as well as to analyze their energy and nutrient intake in order to create nutrition intervention strategies.

All authors included in every chapter are M.D.

In: Focus on Nutrition …
Editor: Teodoro Durá-Travé

ISBN: 978-1-63463-223-2
© 2015 Nova Science Publishers, Inc.

Chapter 1

CATCH-UP ON VERY LOW BIRTH WEIGHT INFANTS

Teodoro Durá-Travé [1,2], *Fidel Gallinas-Victoriano*[2],
Carlos Andrés-Sesma[2], *María García-Ayerra*[2]
and Sada Elena Zarikian-Denis[2]

[1] Department of Pediatrics, Faculty of Medicine,
University of Navarra, Pamplona, Spain
[2] Department of Pediatrics, Navarra Hospital Complex,
Pamplona, Spain

ABSTRACT

Objective. Descriptive anthropometric survey in a cohort of very low birth weight (VLBW) infants from birth to age 8 years, analyzing the growth characteristics in these patients.

Material and Methods. Retrospective record of weight and height at birth and age 0.5, 1, 1.5, 2, 3, 4, 6 and 8 years in a cohort of VLBW infants (<1500 g). Patients were separated into appropriate for gestational age (AGA) and low birth weight or small for gestational age (SGA) according to the charts from Carrascosa et al. Anthropometric variables were compared with those from a control group.

Results. The number of VLBW newborns who were included was 170 (82 males and 88 females): 59.4% (n=101) were AGA and 40.6% (n=69) were SGA. Gestational age was 30.4±3.1 weeks. Weight and height at birth were 1182.1± 228.4 g and 30.5± 3.2 cm, respectively.

Weight, height and body mass index (BMI) in both sexes and every considered age were significantly higher (p<0.05) within the control group with respect to VLBW newborns (AGA and SGA). At age 2, 81.2% and 71% of AGA and SGA (p<0.05) respectively, presented with normal height. At age 8, the height of 8.95% of AGA and 17.4% of SGA infants did not exceed the 2 SD below the average of the control group.

Conclusions. VLBW infants showed catch-up growth, which allows the acquisition of normal height in 87.1% and 78.3% of patients in groups AGA and SGA, respectively, at age 4. Only 8.9% of patients in group AGA did not present catch-up growth at age 8, being the possibility of treatment with growing hormone (GH) not included.

INTRODUCTION

Full-term infants with intrauterine growth restriction are a heterogeneous group with multifactorial conditions that, in addition to present increased perinatal morbidity and mortality, have a higher risk of cardiovascular and/or metabolic disease in adult life [1-3]. These patients show an accelerated compensating growth (catch-up) that is usually complete at age 2 [4-9]. In fact, those patients whose catch-up is not complete have little chance to reach normal stature in adult life. This situation is one of the approved indications to be treated with recombinant growth hormone [10-13].

The increased survival of very low birth weight infants (<1500 g), which is secondary to recent advances in obstetric and perinatal care, entails an increased risk of neurosensory deficits and/or disability [14-16]. Nonetheless, the follow-up of these patients - even with conflicting data - has allowed consideration that their catch-up could even be at a later stage, so conditioning the prognosis of adult size [8, 17-22].

The objective of this chapter is to achieve a longitudinal descriptive study of anthropometric measurements in a cohort of very low birth weight (VLBW) newborn infants, including birth to 8 years of age, and then analyzing the characteristics of catch-up in these patients.

MATERIAL AND METHODS

The institutionalized Program for Child Care in the *Comunidad Foral de Navarra* includes regular health screening that allows the registration of anthropometric measurements (weight and height) in the clinical records, at birth and ages 3, 6, 9, 12, 15, 18 and 24 months and 3, 4, 6, 8, 10, 12 and 14 years.

By means of this infrastructure, the different anthropometric measurements have been recorded (weight and height), and body mass index (Kg/m^2) corresponding to birth and ages 0.5, 1, 1.5, 2, 3, 4, 6 and 8 years has been calculated in a cohort of VLBW infants (< 1500 g). The condition to be included was being Caucasian and a child from Spanish Caucasian parents, born in the Neonatal Unit of the *Complejo Hospitalario de Navarra* within the period January, 2001-December, 2005.

Within this period, 217 births of VLBW infants were recorded, from which 47 cases were excluded for various reasons: perinatal mortality in 20 (9.2%), severe malformations and/or chromosomopathy in 6 (2.8%), severe neurosensory and motor sequelae in 5 (2.3%), ethnic reasons in 8 (3.7%) and other reasons (distance to hospital, lack of continuity in pediatric health screening, etc.) in 8 cases (3.7%).

The entire group of VLBW infants included in the study for this chapter were separated into two different groups: newborns whose weight is appropriate for gestational age (AGA group) and those with low weight for gestational age (SGA group), depending on whether birth weight and/or length were higher or equal/lower than two standard deviations below the average of a reference population for gestational age and sex, respectively. The growth reference charts for newborns applied in this work were those from the *Estudio Transversal Español de Crecimiento* from Carrascosa et al. [23].

On the other side, a group control was obtained from an observational epidemiological study carried out in an infant population (healthy full-term infants, Caucasian and children from Caucasian parents), whose calendar in anthropometric measurements was similar to those for VLBW infants (482 males and 448 females) [24].

An adequate catch-up growth was defined when height in VLBW infants exceeded two standard deviations below the average corresponding to the charts of the control group [4-6].

The results are shown as percentages (%) and means (M) with corresponding standard deviations (SD). The statistical analysis (descriptive statistics, Student's T and comparison of percentages) was calculated by applying the Statistical Packages for the Social Sciences (SPSS) 20.0 program (Chicago, Ill, USA). Statistical significance was assumed when p value was lower than 0.05.

RESULTS

The number of VLBW infants included in this chapter was 170 (82 males and 88 females). Twin pregnancies accounted for 32.4% and multiple pregnancies for 9.4%. Overall, 59.4% (n=101) were preterm infants with appropriate weight for gestational age (AGA group) and the remaining 40.6% (n=69) were preterm infants with low weight for gestational age (SGA group). Within the SGA group, 56.5% of the cases presented with weight and height alterations at birth, whereas exclusive alterations of height (24.4%) or weight (18.8%) were less frequent.

The mean gestational age was 30.4±3.1 weeks (males: 30.4±2.9 and females: 30.5±3.2; NS). Mean values for weight and height were 1182.1 ± 228.4 g (males: 1223.7 ± 208.6 and females: 1143.3 ± 240.3; p<0.05) and 30.5 ± 3.2 cm (males: 38.6 ± 2.8 and females: 37.8 ± 3.5; NS), respectively. Table 1 shows and compares the anthropometric values at birth of the VLBW infants (AGA and SGA groups) for both sexes. There were no statistical differences between mean values for weight and height at birth between both groups. Gestational age was significantly higher in the SGA group than in the AGA group.

Table 1. Anthropometric data from VLBW infants at birth in both sexes

	Males		Females	
	AGA group (n=52) M (SD)	SGA group (n=30) M (SD)	AGA group (n=49) M (SD)	SGA group (n=39) M (SD)
Gestational age	28.67 (1.99)*	33.26 (1.92)*	28.87 (2.12)*	32.64 (3.09)*
Weight (g)	1.204.34** (200.79)	1.257.36** (179.91)	1.145.81** (209.70)	1.140.07** (225.99)
Height (cm)	38.28 (3.07)	39.03 (2.42)	38.20 (2.58)	37.39 (3.45)

(*) p<0.05 among AGA and SGA.
(**) p<0.05 among sexes in the same group.

Table 2 displays and compares the mean values for registered weight and height and calculated BMI for males in every considered age, corresponding to VLBW infants (AGA and SGA groups) and the control group.

Table 2. Average values (males) for weight, height and BMI in VLWB infants (AGA and SGA group) and control group

Weight (kg)			
Age (years)	SGA group M (SD)	AGA group M (SD)	Control group M (SD)
0	1.25 (0.17)	1.20 (0.22)	3.33 (0.44)
0.5	6.06 (0.70)	6.10 (1.01)	7.91 (0.74)
1	8.17 (0.82)	8.45 (1.16)	10.26 (0.94)
1.5	9.03 (1.47)	9.81 (1.81)*	11.69 (1.17)
2	10.03 (1.05)	10.95 (1.53)*	13.02 (1.26)
3	12.53 (1.39)	13.28 (1.92)*	15.34 (1.49)
4	14.61 (2.16)	15.38 (2.30)*	17.75 (2.06)
6	18.71 (3.28)	20.15 (3.47)*	22.60 (3.13)
8	24.30 (4.94)	25.52 (5.28)	28.93 (4.41)
Height (cm)			
Age (years)	SGA group M (SD)	AGA group M (SD)	Control group M (SD)
0	39.03 (2.42)	38.28 (3.07)	50.45 (1.91)
0.5	61.43 (2.80)	60.83 (3.42)	67.86 (2.01)
1	71.56 (2.87)	71.25 (3.74)	76.77 (2.41)
1.5	77.56 (3.07)	79.37 (3.61)*	83.51 (2.65)
2	84.00 (3.30)	85.35 (3.72)*	88.83 (2.99)
3	92.36 (3.69)	93.94 (3.25)*	97.13 (3.18)
4	99.85 (4.15)	101.69 (4.36)*	104.59 (4.10)
6	112.87 (4.94)	115.07 (5.06)*	117.67 (4.84)
8	125.15 (5.77)	127.21 (5.10)*	129.91 (5.53)
BMI (kg/m^2)			
Age (years)	SGA group M (SD)	AGA group M (SD)	Control group M (SD)
0.5	16.05 (1.40)	16.21 (1.56)	17.15 (1.32)
1	15.89 (1.09)	16.19 (1.47)	17.41 (1.30)
1.5	15.38 (1.53)	15.73 (1.45)	16.75 (1.27)
2	14.69 (0.87)	15.06 (1.12)	16.48 (1.14)
3	14.66 (0.95)	14.99 (1.47)	16.24 (1.16)
4	14.59 (1.38)	14.80 (1.39)	16.16 (1.17)
6	14.50 (1.70)	15.10 (1.66)	16.19 (1.44)
8	15.20 (2.08)	15.67 (2.12)	17.09 (1.86)

(*) $p < 0.05$ with respect to the SGA Group.

Mean values for weight, height and BMI were significantly higher ($p < 0.05$) in the control group than in VLBW infants (AGA and SGA groups) in every age considered. Mean values for registered weight at age 1.5, 2, 3, 4 and 6 years were significantly higher ($p < 0.05$) in the AGA group than in the

SGA group. Mean values of registered height at ages 1.5, 2, 3, 4, 6 and 8 years were significantly higher (p<0.05) in the AGA group with respect to the SGA group. However, there were no statistically significant differences among mean values of BMI for every considered age in both groups.

Table 3. Average values (females) for weight, height and BMI in VLBW infants (SGA and AGA groups) and control group

Weight (kg)		
Age (years)	SGA group M (SD)	AGA group M (SD)	Control group M (DE)
0	1.14 (0.25)	1.45 (0.22)*	3.19 (0.38)
0.5	5.04 (0.92)	5.58 (0.75)*	7.39 (0.74)
1	7.19 (1.25)	8.03 (1.03)*	9.61 (1.04)
1.5	8.63 (1.22)	9.62 (1.24)*	11.09 (1.26)
2	9.60 (1.90)	10.72 (1.51)*	12.38 (1.41)
3	11.72 (1.68)	13.02 (2.20)*	14.71 (1.64)
4	14.14 (2.47)	14.97 (2.88)*	16.97 (2.10)
6	18.61 (3.34)	19.69 (3.69)*	21.79 (2.88)
8	24.56 (5.55)	25.54 (5.67)	28.39 (4.48)
Height (cm)		
Age (years)	SGA group M (SD)	AGA group M (SD)	Control group M (SD)
0	37.39 (4.45)	38.20 (2.58)	49.64 (1.80)
0.5	58.94 (4.49)	59.90 (3.34)	66.46 (2.29)
1	69.18 (3.93)	70.92 (3.82)*	75.26 (2.73)
1.5	76.05 (3.71)	77.73 (3.91)*	82.12 (2.88)
2	81.87 (4.16)	83.53 (3.95)*	87.27 (3.07)
3	90.85 (3.77)	92.26 (5.33)*	95.52 (3.36)
4	97.53 (5.17)	99.94 (5.63)*	103.22 (3.99)
6	111.65 (5.64)	113.94 (6.41)	116.53 (4.51)
8	124.15 (5.73)	125.58 (7.15)	128.78 (5.17)
BMI (kg/m^2)		
Age (years)	SGA group M (SD)	AGA group M (SD)	Control group M (SD)
0.5	14.52 (1.83)	15.67 (1.13)*	16.75 (1.29)
1	15.06 (1.39)	16.07 (1.44)*	16.96 (1.57)
1.5	14.91 (1.73)	15.88 (1.08)*	16.38 (1.63)
2	14.28 (2.01)	15.32 (1.19)*	16.24 (1.41)
3	14.15 (1.39)	15.21 (1.43)*	16.09 (1.29)
4	14.48 (1.56)	14.95 (2.51)	15.86 (1.36)
6	14.85 (1.77)	15.06 (1.81)	15.99 (1.45)
8	15.81 (2.41)	16.01 (2.24)	17.06 (1.92)

(*) p<0.05 with respect to the SGA group.

Table 3 outlines and compares the mean values for registered weight and height and calculated BMI in females in every considered age, corresponding to VLBW infants (AGA and SGA groups) and the control group. Mean values for weight, height and BMI were significantly higher (p<0.05) within the control group with respect to VLBW infants (AGA and SGA groups) in every considered age. Mean values for registered weight at birth and ages 0.5, 1, 1.5, 2, 3, 4 and 6 years were significantly higher (p<0.05) within the AGA group than within the SGA group. Mean values for registered height at ages 1, 1.5, 2, 3, 4 and 6 years were significantly higher (p< 0.05) within the AGA group. Finally, mean values for BMI at ages 0.5, 1, 1.5, 2 and 3 years were significantly higher (p<0.05) within the AGA group.

Mean values of the registered weight within the AGA group – in both sexes – overtake the two standard deviations below the mean of the group control at age 1 year, whereas within the SGA group, females did at age 1.5 and males did at age 3 years. Within the AGA group, mean values for registered height did overtake the two standard deviations below the mean of the control group at age 1 year (females) and 1.5 years (males), whereas within the SGA group, they did at age 2 years in both sexes.

Figure 1 sets the percentages of VLBW infants (AGA and SGA groups) whose weights (A) and heights (B) do not overtake the two standard deviations below the mean of the control group in the different ages. Within the AGA group, 81.2% of the cases reached normal (inside the range) height at age 2 years, whereas within the SGA group, 71% (p<0.05) did at that age. In the period of 2-8 years, 9.9% of the cases within the AGA group and 11.6% within the SGA group presented normal height. In this way, at age 8, 8.9% (AGA) and 17.4% (SGA) did not surpass the two standard deviations below the mean of the control group (Note: Two patients in 12 within the SGA group (17.4%) that did not present catch-up at age 8 years initiated treatment with recombinant growth hormone at age 6, and 8 patients did so at age 8 years).

Table 4 provides and compares calculated growth rates (cm/year) in every considered age for both sexes, corresponding to VLBW infants (AGA and SGA) and control group. Within the first 2 years of life, in both sexes, the growth rate in VLBW infants was significantly higher (p<0.05) than in the control group.

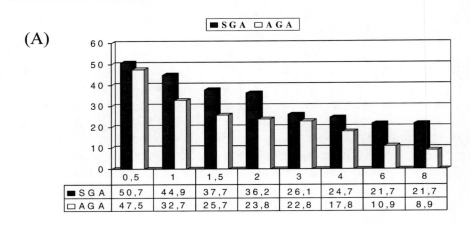

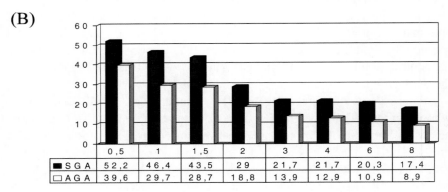

Figure 1. Percentage of VLBW infants (AGA and SGA groups) with subnormal weight (A) and height (B) in the different ages.

Table 4. Growth rate (cm/year) for both sexes in the different groups

Males			
Age (years)	SGA group M (SD)	AGA group M (SD)	Control group M (SD)
1	32.43 (2.72)*	33.48 (2.39)*	26,32 (4,10)
2	12.45 (1.54)*	13.41 (2.00)*	12,06 (1,37)
3	8.49 (1.88)	8.87 (2.16)	8,30 (0,83)
4	7.14 (1.80)	7.24 (1.80)	7,46 (0,74)
6	6.97 (1.58)	6.97 (2.75)	6,54 (0,65)
8	5.96 (1.41)	6.10 (2.25)	6,12 (0,61)

Females			
Age (years)	SGA group M (SD)	AGA group M (SD)	Control group M (SD)
1	31.96 (3.90)*	32.41 (3.16)*	25,62 (4,04)
2	13.08 (1.40)*	12.69 (2.07)*	12,01 (1,36)
3	8.76 (2.38)	8.89 (2.29)	8,25 (0,82)
4	7.65 (2.15)	7.98 (1.61)	7,70 (0,77)
6	5.97 (2.85)	6.44 (2.95)	6,65 (0,66)
8	6.65 (4.94)	6.20 (1.73)	6,12 (0,62)

(*) $p < 0.05$ with respect to the control group.

DISCUSSION

The terms intrauterine growth restriction and small for gestational age (SGA) are not strictly equivalent concepts [25], since they refer to different chronological stages (fetal growth and anthropometric characteristics, respectively); however, they make an allusion to the impossibility of reaching their genetic growth potential during the prenatal period as an adaptive response to an adverse uterine environment. In any case, both terms are used interchangeably to gather those newborns whose weight and/or height at birth are equal/lower than two standard deviations under the mean of an average population, given gestational age and sex. In this particular case, the majority of patients who were included in the so-called SGA group presented alterations in both weight and height at birth, whereas the proportion of patients with exclusive alteration of weight or height was slightly lower.

This definition requires an accurate diagnosis of gestational age and the registration of anthropometric variables after birth, whose values should be compared to specific reference standards for gestational age and sex. The choice of reference standards constitutes a determining factor in the evaluation of the growth of a newborn [26]. In fact, the variability shown in neonatal anthropometric variables in relation to racial, genetic, social, environmental factors and maternal lifestyle makes the use of local and/or national charts advisable. Charts from Lubchenko et al. [27], which were first published in the 1960s, have had a wide circulation and proved clinical usefulness; however, the charts for weight and height in newborns among 26-42 weeks of gestational age from the *Estudio transversal Español de Crecimiento 2008* [23] are more qualified national references at present day.

Fetal development and growth is a complex event in which a harmonious and continuous process of cellular proliferation and differentiation takes place.

Multiple factors (maternal, fetal, placental and environmental) have been described to adversely affect the fetus and trigger a series of functional and structural adaptive changes – it is known as the "thrifty phenotype hypothesis"- that would condition a restriction in fetal growth, as well as a series of changes in hormone sensitivity and/or secretion that would determine a higher risk of presenting metabolic and/or endocrine disorders in adult life [28, 29]. Nevertheless, after birth, some full-term newborns affected with intrauterine growth restriction show an accelerated compensatory growth (*catch-up*), especially during the first year of life, that allows – approximately in 90% of the cases – them to overtake the limit of two standard deviations below the average of a reference population; this means, they reach normal height [4-6, 8, 9]. However, whenever this compensatory growth is not present, they are not likely to have normal height in adult life. This is one of the indications of treatment with growing hormone that has been approved by the *US Food and Drug Administration* (FDA) and the *European Medicines Agency*, with the aim of increasing the initial compensatory growth and/or keeping a normal growth rate [10-13].

Advances in obstetric and/or perinatal care in the past decades have led to substantially reduce the mortality of VLBW infants; however, given the potential sensorineural morbidity, these patients are usually included in follow-up programs for earlier detection of problems in neurocognitive development [14-16]. The optimization of these programs has facilitated the homogeneity in dietary and nutritional recommendations, as well as the possibility to monitor growth in the first years of life. This allows analyzing, as in our chapter, the evolution of anthropometric variables in VLBW infants [30].

The results in this chapter confirm, on one side, that VLBW infants show a compensatory postnatal growth with a maximum peak during the first years of life, as it occurs in full-term small for gestational age infants. In fact, the growth rate during the first 12 months of life in VLBW infants was noticeably higher than that in the control group; this would explain, to a large extent, the high proportion of patients whose height gets into the normal range by the age of 2 years, even showing significant differences between AGA and SGA groups. On the other side, a lower proportion of patients and/or a stunting in catch-up is noticed in VLBW infants with respect to that in full-term small for gestational age infants, since approximately 20% (AGA) and 30% (SGA) of VLBW infants do not exceed two standard deviations below the average of the control group. Nevertheless, around 10% of VLBW infants – in both groups – reach normal height for age and sex between 2 and 8 years of age, and show enough recovery growth in 91.1% (AGA) and 82.6% (SGA) by age 8, respectively.

It should be noted how one in five patients from the SGA group (21.7%) does not get a sufficient rate in catch up by age 4 and, therefore − according to the established European criteria - would be accessible to treatment with growth hormone [6, 8, 9]; and also how one in ten patients from the AGA group (12.9%) do not get a recovery in height by that age, with resulting risk of being short in stature in adult life, being these patients were not accessible to treatment with growth hormone. Therefore, it appears necessary to consider whether the approved criteria for the use of growth hormone in full term small for gestational age infants in the absence of catch-up would be applicable in VLBW infants, since despite being born with adequate for age weight and/or height, the proportion of patients who do not show catch-up by 4 years of age is similar to those full-term small for gestational age infants.

This chapter presents several methodological constraints. As an example, the existence of fetal conditions associated with intrauterine and/or postnatal growth restriction (chromosomal abnormalities, severe malformations, intrauterine infections, etc.) that, in this case, has been a cause of exclusion, has been studied. However, the retrospective nature of this study did not allow us to actively seek maternal socio demographic (age, socio economic and/or educational level, etc.), nutritional or toxic (tobacco, alcohol, psychoactive drugs) conditions that might cause fetal growth restriction, and, occasionally, determine postnatal growth.

As a conclusion, VLBW infants present an accelerated recovery growth, especially in the first 12 months, that helps overtake the two standard deviations under the mean of height - at age 4 - in a reference population in 87.1% (AGA) and 78.3% (SGA) of the patients, respectively. We should remark how the use of growth hormone would not be approved, in the absence of catch-up, in 12.9% of patients at age 4 or 8.9% at age 8 years within the AGA group; this fact should be reconsidered if the approved criteria for the use of growth hormone in full-term small for gestational age infants could also be applied in VLBW infants.

REFERENCES

[1]   Meas T, Deghmoun S, Alberti C, Carreira E, Armoogum P, Chevenne D, et al. Independent effects of weight gain and fetal programming on

metabolic complications in adults born small for gestational age. *Diabetologia* 2010; 53:907-13.

[2]   Whincup PH, Kaye SJ, Owen CG, Huxley R, Cook DG, Anazawa S, et al. Birth weight and risk of type 2 diabetes. A systematic review. *JAMA* 2008; 300: 2886-97.

[3]   Johansson S, Iliadou A, Bergval N, Tuvemo T, Noeman M, Cnattingius S. Risk of high blood pressure among young men increases with the degree of immaturity at birth. *Circulation* 2005; 112:3430-6.

[4]   Lee PA, Chernausek SD, Hokken Koelega ACS, Czernichow P. International Small for gestational age advisory board consensus development conference statement: management of short children born small for gestational age. *Pediatrics* 2003; 111:1253-61.

[5]   Clayton PE, Cianfarani S, Czernichow P, Johannsson G, Rapaport R, Rogol A. Management of the child born small for gestational age through to adulthood: a consensus statement of the International Societies of Pediatric Endocrinology and the Growth Hormone Research Society. *J Clin Endocrinol Metab* 2007;92:804-10.

[6]   Boguszewski MC, Mericq V, Bergada I, Damiani D, Belgorosky A, Gunczler P, Ortiz T, Llano M, Domené HM, Calzada-León R, Blanco A, Barrientos M, Procel P, Lanes R, Jaramillo O. Latin American consensus: children born small for gestational age. *BMC Pediatr* 2011; 11:66.

[7]   Karlberg JP, Albertsson-Wikland K, Kwan EY, Lam BC, Low LC. The timing of early postnatal catch-up growth in normal, full-term infants born short for gestational age. *Horm Res* 1997;48 Suppl 1:17-24.

[8]   Hokken-Koelega AC, De Ridder MA, Lemmen RJ, Den Hartog H, De Muinck Keizer-Schrama SM, Drop SL. Children born small for gestational age: do they catch up? *Pediatr Res* 1995; 38:267-71.

[9]   Karlberg J, Albertsson-Wikland K. Growth in full-term small-for-gestational-age infants: from birth to final height. *Pediatr Res* 1995; 38:733-9.

[10]   Gharib H, Cook DM, Saenger PH, Bengtsson BA, Feld S, Nippold TB, Rodbard HW, Seibel JA, Vance ML, Zimmerman D. American Association of Clinical Endocrinologists Growth Hormone Task Force 2003: American Association of Clinical Endocrinologists medical guidelines for clinical practice for growth hormone use in adults and children–2003 update. *Endocr Pract* 2003, 9:64-73.

[11]   European Agency for the Evaluation of Medicinal Products: Committee for Proprietary Medicinal Products (CPMP) 2003 Norditropin.

[http://www.ema.europa.eu/pdfs/human/referral/norditropin/347803en.p df], Published June 26, 2003. Accessed May 12, 2014.

[12] Argente J, Gracia R, Ibáñez L, Oliver A, Borrajo E, Vela A, López-Siguero JP, Moreno ML, Rodríguez-Hierro F, Spanish SGA Working Group: Improvement in growth after two years of growth hormone therapy in very young children born small for gestational age and without spontaneous catch-up growth: results of a multicenter, controlled, randomized, open clinical trial. *J Clin Endocrinol Metab* 2007, 92:3095-3101.

[13] Carrascosa A, Vicens-Calvet E, Yeste D, Espadero RM, Ulied A. Children born small for gestational age (SGA) who fail to achieve catch up growth by 2-8 years of age are short from infancy to adulthood. Data from a cross-sectional study of 486 Spanish children. *Pediatr Endocrinol Rev* 2006; 4:15-27.

[14] Lemons JA, Bauer CR, Oh W, Korones SB, Papile LA, Stoll BJ, Verter J, Temprosa M, Wright LL, Ehrenkranz RA, Fanaroff AA, Stark A, Carlo W, Tyson JE, Donovan EF, Shankaran S, Stevenson DK. Very low birth weight outcomes of the National Institute of Child health and human development neonatal research network, January 1995 through December 1996. NICHD Neonatal Research Network. *Pediatrics* 2001; 107:E1.

[15] Arce Casas A, Iriondo Sanz M, Krauel Vidal J, Jiménez González R, Campistol Plana J, Poo Argüelles P, Ibáñez M. Neurological follow-up of very low birth weight newborns at the age of two years (1998-1999). *An Pediatr* (Barc) 2003; 59:454-61.

[16] Hernández González N, Salas Hernández S, García-Alix Pérez A, Roche Herrero C, Pérez Rodríguez J, Omeñaca Teres F, Quero Jiménez J. Morbidity at 2 years in infants with a birth weight of < 1,500 g. *An Pediatr* (Barc) 2005; 62:320-7.

[17] Saigal S, Stoskopf BL, Streiner DL, Burrows E. Physical growth and current health status of infants who were of extremely low birth weight and controls at adolescence. *Pediatrics* 2001; 108:407-15.

[18] Hack M, Schluchter M, Cartar L, Rahman M, Cuttler L, Borawski E. Growth of very low birth weight infants to age 20 years. *Pediatrics* 2003; 112:e30-8.

[19] Finken MJ, Dekker FW, de Zegher F, Wit JM. Long-term height gain of prematurely born children with neonatal growth restraint: parallellism with the growth pattern of short children born small for gestational age. *Pediatrics* 2006; 118:640-3.

[20] Hack M, Flannery D, Schlutcher M, Cartar L, Borawski E, Klein N. outcomes in young adulthood for very low birth weight infants. N Engl J Med 2002;346:149-157.

[21] Niklasson A, Engstrom E, Hard AL, Albertsson-Wikland K, Hellstrom A. Growth in very preterm children: a longitudinal study. *Pediatr Res* 2003;54:899–905

[22] Farooqi A, Hägglöf B, Sedin G, Gothefors L, Serenius F. Growth in 10- to 12-year-old children born at 23 to 25 weeks' gestation in the 1990s: a Swedish national prospective follow-up study. *Pediatrics* 2006; 118:e1452-65.

[23] Carrascosa A, Fernández JM, Fernández C, Ferrández A, López-Siguero JP, Sánchez E, Grupo Colaborador Español, et al. Spanish cross-sectional growth study 2008. Height, weight and body mass index values from birth to adulthood. *An Pediatr* (Barc) 2008; 68:552–69.

[24] Durá Travé T, Garralda Torres I, Hualde Olascoaga J; Grupo Colaborador de Navarra. Longitudinal study of child growth in Navarre (1993-2007). *An Pediatr* (Barc) 2009; 70:526-33.

[25] Wit JM, Finken MJJ, Rijken M, De Zegher F. Preterm growth restraint: A paradigm that unifies intrauterine growth retardation and preterm extrauterine growth retardation and has Implications for the small-for-gestational-age indication in growth hormone therapy. *Pediatrics* 2006; 117:e793-795.

[26] Ayerza Casas A, Rodríguez Martínez G, Samper Villagrasa MP, Ventura Faci P. To born small for gestational age may depend on the growth curve used. *Nutr Hosp* 2011; 26:752-8.

[27] Lubchenco LO, Hansman C, Boyd E. Intrauterine growth in length and head circumference as estimated from live births at gestational ages from 26 to 42 weeks. *Pediatrics* 1966; 47: 403-8.

[28] Hales CN, Barker DJP. The thrifty phenotype hypothesis. *Br Med Bull* 2001; 60:5-20.

[29] Fall CHD. Endocrine programming and the fetal and early-life origins of adult disease. In: Clinical Pediatrics Endocrinology. Brook Ch, Clayton P, Brown, eds. *Blackwell Publishing. Massachusetts, USA.* 2005. pp.396-409.

[30] López ID, Muñoz Ade A, Muñoz JB, Rodríguez PC, Gómez EG, Ollero MJ, Rodríguez JM, Dehlia AC, Estrada RC, Toda LI. Follow-up of the small-for-gestational-age child: clinical guidelines. *An Pediatr (Barc)* 2012; 76:104.e1-7

In: Focus on Nutrition …
Editor: Teodoro Durá-Travé

ISBN: 978-1-63463-223-2
© 2015 Nova Science Publishers, Inc.

Chapter 2

ADHERENCE TO MEDITERRANEAN DIET IN STUDENTS OF COMPULSORY SECONDARY EDUCATION (13-16 YEARS)

Teodoro Durá-Travé[1,2], Fidel Gallinas-Victoriano[2], Arantxa Mosquera-Gorostidi[2], Abel Justo-Ranera[2] and Isabel San Martín-García[2]

[1] Department of Pediatrics, Faculty of Medicine,
University of Navarra, Pamplona, Spain
[2] Department of Pediatrics, Navarra Hospital Complex, Pamplona, Spain

ABSTRACT

Objective. Mediterranean diet is considered as a prototype of healthy diet. The modernization of society implies sociological and cultural changes that affect feeding preferences and habits. The aim of this chapter is to determine the dietary quality index in students of compulsory secondary education (CSE).

Material and methods. Data collection after distributing a 16 item questionnaire (Kidmed test) to a random sample of 1956 students of CSE (966 males and 990 females): the final score of Kidmed index (range 0-12) indicates whether the degree of adherence to Mediterranean diet is low (0-3), medium (4-7) or high (8-12).

Results. A low Kidmed index value was registered in 6.7% of the students of CSE, whereas medium values corresponded to 50.4% and low values to 42.9%, showing no significant statistical differences among sexes. The Kidmed index decreases progressively with age (p< 0.05). At age 13 (first grade of CSE), 49.5% of the students had an optimal score of Kidmed index, whereas this score reached 37.2% at age 16 (fourth grade of CSE). There were statistical differences (p< 0.05) regarding consumption of fruits, fish, nuts and dried food, sweets and factory produced baked goods, as well as frequency of the absence of breakfast and the attendance to fast food restaurants.

Conclusions. By the end of CSE (at 16 years old), 62.8% of students showed low-medium degree of adherence to Mediterranean diet. Applicable food advices for these adolescents would be increasing consumption of fruits, vegetables, nuts, pasta and rice, yogurt and cheese, legumes and fish, and olive oil as culinary fat; and decreasing consumption of factory produced baked goods and sweets and frequency of fast food restaurants, in addition to insisting on the importance of daily breakfast. In addition, it would be convenient to develop nutrition education programs during compulsory education.

INTRODUCTION

The dietary pattern that has been traditionally observed in Mediterranean countries has given rise to the concept of Mediterranean Diet, characterized by a frequent consumption of vegetables, legumes, fruits, nuts and cereals and, especially, olive oil, as well as a moderate intake of fish, eggs and dairy products (mainly yogurt or cheese), and low intake of animal meat and fat [1-4]. The Mediterranean Diet is considered as a prototype of healthy diet, since it ensures an appropriate calorie and nutrients intake (sufficient amount and adequate proportions) [5-8]; in addition, it contributes to the prevention of cardiovascular disease, hypertension, diabetes, cancer, etc. and, overall, a higher life expectancy [4, 9-14].

The modernization of society entails a series of cultural and sociological changes that inevitably affects feeding habits and preferences. We dedicate less and less time every day to buy and elaborate healthy dishes, as we have an obvious alternative: processed food "easy to cook and fast to eat", which usually brings about an excessive intake of food from animal origin, especially meat and derivatives, and refined sugar, with its consequent increase in saturated fat (SFA) and cholesterol in the diet [8, 15-19].

This deterioration of traditional eating patterns in our population takes place especially in those sectors more likely to be influenced by the environment such as, for example, children and adolescents [16, 20-23]. In addition, these are the sectors that most need healthy feeding for optimal growing and development. Therefore, adolescent population constitutes a nutritional group at risk that would justify the study of the quality of feeding habits.

The purpose of this chapter is to determine the quality index of the dietary habits (adherence to Mediterranean diet) among the students of compulsory secondary education in the city of Pamplona.

MATERIAL AND METHODS

The city of Pamplona comprises a total population of 183.964 inhabitants (National Institute of Statistics, Spain), of which 6179 (3.36%) constitute the group of population with ages among 13 to 16 years and/or students of compulsory secondary education (CSE) in the year 2007. The sampling frame considered is this group of 6179 adolescents (3145 males and 3034 females). The most unfavorable hypothesis (0.50), a 99% confidence level (α=0.01) and an accuracy of 0.03 has been taken in order to calculate the sample size, being the minimum number of individuals necessary 1419 students [24].

The *Test de Adhesión a la Dieta Mediterránea Kidmed* has been successfully applied in this group of population in order to assess the quality of feeding habits (adherence to a Mediterranean dietary pattern) [25, 26]. The sample has been obtained by distributing a questionnaire (Kidmed test) to all the CSE students of a random selection of six public or subsidized centers in Pamplona, in a school day within the second trimester of the academic year 2007-2008. Every student who had attended the different academic centers the day fixed for the distribution of the questionnaire (n=1980) accepted to participate; however, 25 questionnaires were rejected owing to incomplete or wrong fulfillment. Therefore, the participation rate could be considered to be 98.8%.

The total number of participants was 1956 students: 966 males (49.4%) and 990 females (50.6%). The distribution by grade and sex was: 1º CSE (n=517), 256 males and 261 females; 2º CSE (n=530), 260 males and 270 females; 3º CSE (n=447), 240 males and 207 females, and 4º CSE (n=462), 210 males and 252 females. The comparison of proportions among the different grades of CSE applied a beta risk of 0.01 (99% power).

The Kidmed test (table 1) is a 16 item questionnaire that has to be answered either as an affirmative or negative way (yes/no). The affirmative answers in those questions representing a negative connotation of

Mediterranean diet (4 questions) count as -1 point, whereas the affirmative answers in those questions that include a positive aspect with regards to Mediterranean diet (12 questions) count as +1 point. Negative answers do not count. Therefore, the index can range from 0 (minimum adherence) to 12 (maximum adherence).

The sum of the values of this questionnaire results in the KIDMED index, which is classified into three categories:

a)   8 to 12: Optimal Mediterranean diet (high level of adherence)
b)   4 to 7: need to improve dietary habits to adjust to Mediterranean pattern (medium level of adherence)
c)   0 to 3: low quality diet (low level of adherence)

The results are displayed as percentages. Statistical analysis (chi-square test) was performed using the SPSS 17.0 for Windows software package.

Table 1. KIDMED test to assess the Mediterranean Diet

KIDMED test Scoring	
Takes a fruit or fruit juice every day	+1
Has a second piece of fruit every day	+1
Has fresh or cooked vegetables regularly once a day	+1
Has fresh or cooked vegetables more than once a day	+1
Consumes fish regularly (at least 2–3/week)	+1
Goes >1/ week to a fast food restaurant (hamburger)	-1
Likes legumes and eats them >1/week	+1
Consumes pasta or rice almost every day (5 or more per week)	+1
Has cereals or grains (bread, etc) for breakfast	+1
Consumes nuts regularly (at least 2–3/week)	+1
Uses olive oil at home	+1
Skips breakfast some days	-1
Has a dairy product for breakfast (yoghurt, milk, etc)	+1
Has commercially baked goods or pastries for breakfast	-1
Takes two yoghurts and/or some cheese (40 g) daily	+1
Takes sweets and candy several times every day	-1

RESULTS

Table 2 outlines and presents a comparison of the results of the Kidmed test for both sexes. A low value for the Kidmed test was registered in 6.7% of the entire sample, whereas medium value in 50.4% and high value in 42.9%, showing no significant differences between sexes. However, there are statistically significant differences ($p<0.05$) among different items: males attend a fast food restaurant once or more a week, eat pasta or rice almost on a daily basis (5 or more times a week), have cereals or derivatives (bread, toasts, etc.) at breakfast, eat nuts at least 2 or 3 times a week and have industrial pastries for breakfast more frequently than females; females have fresh or cooked vegetables once a day and do not have breakfast everyday more frequently than males.

Table 3 lists and compares the results of the Kidmed test according to grade and/or age, noting a progressive decrease in the Kidmed index with age. At age 13, (1st grade CSE), 49.5% of individuals have an optimal assessment of Kidmed index, whereas at age 16 (4th grade CSE), this optimal assessment was 37.2%. There were significant differences ($p<0.05$) among students of 1st grade and 4th grade in the following items: daily consumption of a second fruit (44.15 vs. 32%), fish at least 2 or 3 times a week (73.5% vs. 68.7%), nuts at least 2 or 3 times a week (43.3% vs. 38.5%), industrial pastries for breakfast (15.1% vs. 22.5%) and sweets several times a day (13% vs. 19.5%), as well as in a skipping breakfast (12.2% vs. 17.1%) and the attendance to fast food restaurants (6.4% vs. 10.4%).

Table 2. Mediterranean diet quality index in CSE students according to sex

KIDMED test	Males (%)	Females (%)	Total (%)
Takes a fruit or fruit juice every day	81.6	83.5	82.6
Has a second piece of fruit every day	38.9	40.6	39.8
Has fresh or cooked vegetables regularly once a day (*)	74.5	79.9	77.2
Has fresh or cooked vegetables more than once a day	26.2	27.3	26.7
Consumes fish regularly (at least 2–3/week)	66.4	66.7	66.5

Table 2. (Continued)

KIDMED test	Males (%)	Females (%)	Total (%)
Goes >1/ week to a fast food restaurant (hamburger) (*)	12.0	7.7	9.8
Likes legumes and eats them >1/week	74.4	72.8	73.6
Consumes pasta or rice almost every day (5 or more per week) (*)	46.8	36.3	41.5
Has cereals or grains (bread, etc) for breakfast (*)	79.6	73.3	76.4
Consumes nuts regularly (at least 2–3/week) (*)	45.7	34.3	39.9
Uses olive oil at home	72.5	73.8	73.2
Skips breakfast some days (*)	13.0	21.5	17.3
Has a dairy product for breakfast (yoghurt, milk, etc)	90.9	88.8	89.8
Has commercially baked goods or pastries for breakfast (*)	23.1	15.1	19.0
Takes two yoghurts and/or some cheese (40 g) daily	53.1	51.7	52.4
Takes sweets and candy several times every day	18.3	16.5	17.4
KIDMED Index			
<3	6.3	7.2	6.7
4-7	49.5	51.1	50.4
>8	44.2	41.7	42.9

(*) $p < 0.05$ (Chi-square).

Table 3. Mediterranean diet quality index in CSE students according to academic grade

KIDMED test	1° CSE (%)	2° CSE (%)	3° CSE (%)	4° CSE (%)
Takes a fruit or fruit juice every day	84.1	81.7	83.7	80.7
Has a second piece of fruit every day (*)	44.1	42.5	39.6	32.0
Has fresh or cooked vegetables regularly once a day	80.7	75.5	76.5	76.2
Has fresh or cooked vegetables more than once a day	27.5	29.2	22.8	26.8

KIDMED test	1° CSE (%)	2° CSE (%)	3° CSE (%)	4° CSE (%)
Consumes fish regularly (at least 2–3/week) (*)	73.5	67.5	65.3	58.7
Goes >1/ week to a fast food restaurant (hamburger) (*)	6.4	12.1	10.5	10.4
Likes pulses and eats them >1/week	74.7	68.5	75.4	76.6
Consumes pasta or rice almost every day (5 or more per week)	41.5	44.5	43.4	39.6
Has cereals or grains (bread, etc) for breakfast	78.1	78.3	73.6	75.1
Consumes nuts regularly (at least 2–3/week) (*)	43.3	41.9	35.1	38.5
Uses olive oil at home	73.8	72.8	72.6	73.5
Skips breakfast some days (*)	12.2	20.6	19.7	17.1
Has a dairy product for breakfast (yoghurt, milk, etc)	90.5	88.9	89.3	90.7
Has commercially baked goods or pastries for breakfast (*)	15.1	19.8	19.0	22.5
Takes two yoghurts and/or some cheese (40 g) daily	55.1	50.2	50.1	54.1
Takes sweets and candy several times every day (*)	13.0	19.8	17.4	19.5
KIDMED Index				
<3	4.8	8.3	7.4	6.5
4-7	45.7	46.4	54.1	56.3
>8	49.5	45.3	38.5	37.2

(*) $p < 0.05$ (Chi-square)

DISCUSSION

Different assessment scales have been developed in the past so as to evaluate the adherence to Mediterranean diet; they are usually based on qualitative and/or quantitative aspects of the intake of the different "typical" components of Mediterranean diet [7, 18, 27-30]. These quality indexes of Mediterranean diet have been applied mainly in adult populations and require a laborious and complex processing of the collected information on food consumption. At present day, the Kidmed test is available and is easy to fulfill by the survey respondent and easy to interpret by the survey taker. This test has been made on the basis of the previously cited indexes and/or principles that support the Mediterranean diet, but it is adapted to the pediatric age and allows a quick assessment of the quality of feeding habits and, in particular, a determination of the adherence level to Mediterranean diet[25]. The Kidmed

Index constitutes an instrument that, on one side, allows a quick identification of populations with unhealthy feeding habits and, on the other side, has proved that a higher score guarantees a supply of nutrients in sufficient amount and adequate proportions, being this one of the reasons that justifies its use [31].

The analysis of the answers to the different items discloses that only 42.9% of surveyed students follow feeding habits compatible with the Mediterranean dietary pattern (high level of adherence). This means, most of the students of CSE (the remaining 57.1%) show medium or low level of adherence and, therefore, the need to improve their feeding habits in order to adjust them to the Mediterranean standards. Overall, it is remarkable how the surveyed adolescents do not fulfill the recommendations of food intake for the majority of foods that make up the base of the food pyramid; this means, fruits (barely 39.8% had a second piece of fruit daily), vegetables (26.7% refer to have a second serving daily), nuts (hardly 39.9% eat nuts during the week) and pasta or rice (41.5% eat them on a daily basis). In addition, the intake of yogurt and cheese was also proportionally low. On the other hand, it should also be emphasized the relatively high percentage of adolescents that have industrial pastries for breakfast (19% of students) or have sweets every day (17.4%); we should note that these foods are on top of the food pyramid and, therefore, their consumption should be occasional. The Mediterranean diet represents, besides a healthy diet, a lifestyle that is confined to a specific climate and geographic area [2-5, 18]; in this sense, the trend to frequent fast food restaurants in adolescents (9.8% of the respondents go once or even more a week) and/or and the omission of breakfast (17.3% of respondents do not have breakfast daily) denote, to a great extent, a loss of cultural heritage that Mediterranean diet represents. Olive oil is an essential component of Mediterranean culture that unswervingly prevails in the different ethnic groups or current Mediterranean countries and, a largely responsible for the beneficial effects that have been attributed to this dietary pattern [4, 32]. This explains, in large measure, why the culinary consumption of olive oil at home is majorly referred by the respondents [18, 19].

The analysis of the Kidmed index in relation to age and/or grade displays a progressive deterioration in the adherence to Mediterranean diet: whereas 49.5% of students of 1st grade obtain an optimal score in the test (high level of adherence), barely 37.2% of the students of 4th grade get that score. This decline −essentially due to a lower intake of fruits and vegetables, fishes and nuts and a higher intake of industrial pastries and sweets, as well as a low consistency in breakfast and a high frequency of fast food consumption- highlights a trend in CSE students to join the new occidental feeding pattern, which includes an increasing production and consumption of processed food at the expense of Mediterranean cooking, based on a wide variety of fresh and natural food. By the end of compulsory education, 62.8% of students – no differences among sexes- manifest a low-medium adherence to Mediterranean diet as a consequence of the progressive loss of traditional dietary habits of our geographical environment. On one hand, this fact allows considering that a high rate of adolescents have some risk of suffering from nutritional deficiency and/or imbalance [26] and, on the other hand, raises concerns regarding a virtual disappearance of the Mediterranean diet in the short to medium term [23, 33, 34].

The results from this chapter illustrate the need for a nutritional education in general population, and more specifically adolescents. Adolescents should learn that Mediterranean diet, as a standard of healthy feeding, contributes to maintain an optimal health status and that, even when it includes all kind of food, the frequency of consumption must follow the lines indicated in the food pyramid. Therefore, the dietary standards applicable to adolescents would consist basically in increasing daily intake of fresh fruit, fresh and/or raw vegetables, pasta and/or rice, nuts (hazelnuts, almonds, walnuts, peanuts, pine nuts, etc.), milk and derivatives, mainly yogurt and cheese, as well as legumes and fish at least 2 or 3 times a week; in addition, the use of olive oil as the only culinary fat should be encouraged. On the other hand, the consumption of industrial pastries and sweets should be recommended as occasional, and daily breakfast including cereals, dairy products and fruits should be emphasized [35, 36]. Nevertheless, we should advise that this chapter has several methodological constraints, since the anthropometric variables and lifestyles (familiar socio-economic status and/or educational qualifications, physical exercise, television watching habits, etc.) of the respondents were not registered, and they could condition, to some extent, the level of adherence to Mediterranean diet [18, 29].

To sum up, it would be useful to develop nutritional education programs that, taking into account the social and familiar context, aim at getting that adolescents be able to carry out healthy feeding. In order to do so, the public institutions should coordinate enough human or material resources to try to maintain our traditional feeding habits and make them compatible with the new lifestyles of modern societies, promoting the dietary counseling in the programs of primary care and developing nutrition and feeding programs in formal education, so that whenever adolescents finish compulsory education, they have an excellent tool to prevent disease and promote health.

REFERENCES

[1]   Helsing E. Traditional diets and disease patterns of the Mediterranean, circa 1960. *Am J Clin Nutr* 1995; 61 (Suppl):1329-1337.

[2]   Willet WC, Sacks F, Trichopoulou A, Drescher G, Ferro-Luzzi A, Helsing E y Trichoupoulos D. Mediterranean diet pyramid: a cultural model for healthy eating. *Am J Clin Nutr* 1995; 61 (Suppl):1402-1406.

[3]   Trichopoulou A y Lagiou P. Healthy traditional Mediterranean diet: an expression of culture, history, and lifestyle. *Nutr Rev* 1997; 55:383-9

[4]   Díaz I, Gascón E, Lázaro S y Maximiano C. Guía de la Alimentación Mediterránea. Ed. Empresa Pública Desarrollo Agrario y Pesquero. Consejería de Agricultura y Pesca. *Junta de Andalucía.* 2007.

[5]   Sánchez-Villegas A, Bes-Rastrollo M, Martínez-González y JA,Serra-Majem L. Adherence to a Mediterranean dietary pattern and weight gain in a follow-up study: the SUN cohort. *Int J Obes* 2006; 30:350-358.

[6]   Hu FB (2003) The Mediterranean diet and mortality – olive oil and beyond. *New Engl J Med* 348, 2595–2596.

[7]   Trichopoulou A, Costacou T, Christina B y Trichopoulou D. Adherence to a Mediterranean diet and survival in a Greek population. *New Engl J Med* 2003; 348:2599–2608.

[8]   Tur JA, Serra-Majem L, Romaguera D y Pous A. Does the diet of the Balearic population, a Mediterranean type diet, still provide adequate antioxidant nutrient intakes? *Eur J Nutr* 2005, 44:204-213.

[9]   Kris-Etherton P, Eckel RH, Howard BV, St Jeor S y Bazarre TL. Lyon Diet Heart Study. Benefits of a Mediterranean-style, national cholesterol education program/American Heart Association step I dietary pattern on cardiovascular disease. *Circulation* 2001; 103: 1823–1825.

[10]   Ferrara LA, Raimondi S, d'Episcopo L, Guilda L, Dello Russo A y Marotta T. Olive oil and reduced need for antihypertensive medications. *Arch Intern Med* 2000; 160:837–842.

[11]   Estruch R, Martínez-González MA, Corella D, Salas-Salvadó J, Ruiz-Gutiérrez V, Covas MI, Fiol M, Gómez-Gracia E, López-Sabater MC, Vinyoles E, Arós F, Conde M, Lahoz C, Lapetra J, Sáez G y Ros E. PREDIMED Study Investigators. Effects of a Mediterranean-style diet on cardiovascular risk factors: a randomized trial. *Ann Intern Med* 2006; 145:1-11.

[12]   Hu FB, Rimm EB, Stampfer MJ, Ascherio A, Spiegelman D y Willet WC. Prospective study of major dietary patterns and risk of coronary heart disease in men. *Am J Clin Nutr* 2000; 72:912-21.

[13] Terry P, Hu FB, Hansen H y Wolk A. Prospective study of major dietary patterns and colorectal risk in women. *Am J Epidemiol* 2001; 154:1143-9.

[14] Trichopoulou A, Naska A, Antoniou A, Friel S, Trygg K y Turrini A. Vegetable and fruit: the evidence in their favour and the public health perspective. *Int J Vitam Nutr Res* 2003; 73:63-9.

[15] Rodríguez F, Banegas JR, Graciani MA, Hernández R y Rey J. Food and nutrient consumption in Spain in the period 1940-1988. Analysis of its consistency with the Mediterranean diet. *Med Clin* (Barc) 1996; 106:161-168.

[16] Durá T. Energy and nutrient intake in compulsory high school students. *An Esp Pediatr* 2001; 54:547-554.

[17] Aranceta J. Spanish food patterns. *Public Health Nutr* 2001; 4:1399–1402.

[18] Sánchez-Villegas A, Martinez JA, De Irala I y Martinez-González MA. Determinants of the adherence to an "a priori" defined Mediterranean dietary pattern. *Eur J Nutr* 2002; 41:249-257.

[19] Moreno LA, Sarría A y Popkin BM. The nutrition transition in Spain: a European Mediterranean country. *Eur J Clin Nutr* 2002; 56:992–1003.

[20] Iturbe A, Emparanza J y Perales A. Dietary pattern of adolescents in Guipuzcoa. *An Esp Pediatr* 1999; 50:471-478.

[21] Samuelson G, Bratteby LE, Enghardt H y Hedgren M. Food habits and energy and nutrient in Swedish adolescents approaching the year 2000. *Acta Paediatr* 1996 (Suppl 415):1-20.

[22] Serra-Majem L, García-Closas R, Ribas L, Carmen Pérez-Rodrigo C y Aranceta J. Food patterns of Spanish schoolchildren and adolescents: The enKid Study. *Public Health Nutrition* 2001; 4:1433-1438.

[23] Tur JA, Romaguera D y Pons A. Food consumption patterns in a mediterranean region: does the mediterranean diet still exist? *Ann Nutr Metab.* 2004;48(3):193-201.

[24] Fernández P. Determination of sample size. Cad Aten Primaria 1996; 3: 138-41 (updated 06/03/2001). Available at URL: http://www.fisterra.com

[25] Serra-Majem L, Ribas L, Ngo J, Ortega RM, García A, Pérez-Rodrigo C y Aranceta J. Food, Youth and the Mediterranean diet in Spain. Development of KIDMED, Mediterranean Diet Quality Index in children and adolescents. *Public Health Nutrition.* 2004; 7: 931-935.

[26] Martínez MI, Hernández MD, Ojeda M, Mena R, Alegre A, Alfonso JL. Development of a program of nutritional education and valuation of the

change of healthful nourishing habits in a population of students of Obligatory Secondary Education. *Nutr Hosp* 2009; 24:504-510.

[27]   Kim S, Haines PS, Siega-Riz AM y Popkin BM. The Diet Quality Index-International (DQI-I) provides an effective tool for cross-national comparison of diet quality as illustrated by China and the United States. *J Nutr* 2003; 133: 3476–3484.

[28]   Tur JA, Romaguera D y Pons A. The Diet Quality Index-International (DQI-I): is it a useful tool to evaluate the quality of the Mediterranean diet?. *Br J Nutr* 2005; 93: 369–376.

[29]   González CA, Argilaga S, Agudo A, Amiano P, Barricarte A, Beguiristain JM, Chirlaque MD, Dorronsoro M, Martinez C, Navarro C, Quirós JR, Rodriguez M y Tormo MJ. Sociodemographic differences in adherence to the Mediterranean dietary pattern in Spanish populations. *Gac Sanit* 2002; 16: 214–221.

[30]   Tur JA, Romaguera D y Pons A. Adherence to the Mediterranean dietary pattern among the population of the Balearic Islands. *Br J Nutr* 2004; 92:341–346.

[31]   Serra-Majem LI, Ribas L, García A, Pérez-Rodrigo C y Aranceta J. Nutrient adequacy and Mediterranean Diet in Spanish school children and adolescents. *Eur J Clin Nutr* 2003; 57 (Suppl 1):S35-S39.

[32]   López J, Gómez P, Castro P, Marín C, Paz E, Bravo MD, Blanco J, Jiménez J, Fuentes F y Pérez F. Mediterranean diet improves low density lipoprotein susceptibility to oxidative modifications. *Med Clin* (Barc) 2000; 115: 361-365.

[33]   Guerra A, Feldl F y Koletzko B. Fatty acid composition of plasma lipids in healthy Portuguese children: is the Mediterranean diet disappearing? *Ann Nutr Metab* 2001; 45:78–81.

[34]   Schmidhuber J. The European Diet – Evolution, Evaluation and Impacts of the CAP. *Organización de las Naciones Unidas para la Agricultura y la Alimentación (FAO).* 2008.

[35]   Nicklas TA, Reger C, Myers y O'Neil C: Breakfast consumption with and without vitamin-mineral supplement use favourably impacts daily nutrient intake of ninth-grade students. *J Adolesc Health* 2000; 27:314-321.

[36]   Durá T. Breakfast among students of compulsory secondary education. *Nutr Hosp* 2002; 17:189-196.

In: Focus on Nutrition …
Editor: Teodoro Durá-Travé

ISBN: 978-1-63463-223-2
© 2015 Nova Science Publishers, Inc.

Chapter 3

NATURAL EVOLUTION OF EXCESS BODY WEIGHT (OVERWEIGHT AND OBESITY) IN CHILDREN

Teodoro Durá-Travé[1,2], Fidel Gallinas-Victoriano[2],
Noelia Ulibarrena-Ascarza[2],
Izaskun Naberán-Mardaras[2],
Ana Amézqueta-Tiraplegui[2]
and Ana Navedo de las Heras[1]
[1]Department of Pediatrics, Faculty of Medicine, University
of Navarra, Pamplona, Spain
[2]Department of Pediatrics, Navarra Hospital Complex, Pamplona, Spain

ABSTRACT

Objective. To analyze the chronological evolution of excess body weight (overweight and obesity) in order to raise public awareness within the different areas of intervention (family, school, business environment, health services) to develop effective measures.

Material and methods. Weight, height and body mass index (BMI) of 604 healthy subjects (307 males and 297 females) have been recorded at birth and ages 1, 2, 3, 4, 6, 8, 10, 12 and 14 years. The presence of excess body weight has been calculated by applying the national references from Ferrández et al.

Results. The prevalence of excess body weight at age 14 years was significantly higher ($p<0.05$) in males (29%) than in females (12.8%). BMI (kg/m^2) was significantly higher ($p<0.05$) in both sexes in every period of age, except for birth and age 1 year, in those patients with excess body weight at age 14, with respect to patients with normal nutritional status of the same age. Those groups with excess body weight at age 14 presented BMI (Z-score) reaching overweight or obesity levels at age 4, and progressively increasing.

Conclusions. Excess body weight would appear at early stages in life, when children's dietary habits depend almost exclusively on family habits, and would increase in the course of school attendance. Finally, a disproportionate weight increase occurs in adolescence probably in relation to unhealthy dietary habits and lifestyles.

INTRODUCTION

The prevalence of excess body weight in childhood (overweight and obesity) has gradually increased in industrialized countries, representing, at present day, the most relevant nutrition disorder in our environment [1-4]. In addition, it should be considered that an excess body weight at any pediatric age, specially in school age, represents a high risk situation for overweight/obesity in adolescence [5-9], and the fact that the majority of adolescents with excess weight will stay in the same condition in adult age, presenting an additional risk of higher levels of morbidity and mortality [10-12].

The World Health Organization (WHO) considers this condition as a major public health problem [13], given its labor, social, economic and sanitary impact. Within this context, the *Estrategia para la Nutrición, Actividad Física y Prevención de la Obesidad (NAOS)* [14], a Spanish strategy for nutrition, physical activity and prevention of obesity, was designed in our country in order to support initiatives that contribute to achieve the necessary social change required to reverse the trend towards excess body weight. This strategic plan gives priority to the prevention of excess body weight in the pediatric age and, in addition, it proposes the creation of an *Obesity Observatory* for the evaluation and monitoring of concrete steps to be adopted in the different areas of assistance (family, school, corporate and sanitary environment). Our community does not have a program for prevention of childhood obesity that includes specialized care as a checker of the necessary methodological consistency in the prevention and treatment of this disease.

Therefore, this situation allows us to propose the possibility of studying the "natural evolution" of excess body weight.

The objective of this chapter is to analyze the chronological evolution of excess body weight in our environment, and, in this way, to raise awareness in the different areas of intervention referred by the NAOS strategy to assume appropriate measures in each moment.

MATERIAL AND METHODS

An observational, longitudinal study carried out in an infant population (Caucasian healthy individuals, and the children of Caucasian parents from Spanish origin), whose methodology has been explained in detail in previous issues [8, 15], has permitted the extraction of 604 healthy individuals aged 14 years (307 males and 297 females). These patients were attended according to the Healthcare Screening Program for pediatric population of the Community of Navarre [16] in 2007, and their anthropometric data (weight and height) were collected and registered in their respective medical records. In the same way, the anthropometric data (weight and height) for each individual corresponding to birth and ages 1, 2, 3, 4, 6, 8, 10 and 12 years was retrospectively obtained.

Body mass index (BMI) has been calculated by using the following formula: weight (kg)/height^2 (m). The Z-score values for BMI were determined using the SEINAPTRACKER program (Medicalsoft Intercath, S.L. University of Barcelona, 2007-2008), being the charts and growing curves from Ferrández et al. (Centro Andrea Prader, Zaragoza 2002) [17] the reference patterns. BMI (Z-score) values of +1.0 (85th percentile) and +2.0 (97th percentile) were established as cut points in order to define overweight and obesity. In addition, the prevalence of excess body weight (overweight and obesity) at age 14 years has been determined by applying the international references from Cole et al. [18], which set BMI cut points (kg/m^2) to define overweight and obesity by extrapolation of adult values proposed by the WHO (25 and 30 kg/m^2 respectively). Patients were placed in three different groups: standard group (normal nutrition at age 14), overweight group (overweight at age 14) and obesity group (obesity at age 14).

Results are expressed as percentages (%) and means (M) with corresponding standard deviations (SD). Statistical analysis (descriptive statistics, Student's T-Test, Chi-square Test) was performed using the *Statistical Packages for the Social Sciences* (SPSS) software, version 20.0

(Chicago, Illinois, USA). Statistical significance level was reported when p value was lower than 0.05.

RESULTS

Table 1 shows and compares the prevalence of excess body weight (overweight and obesity) at age 14 years in both sexes according to the references used. There were not any statistically significant differences in prevalence of excess body weight regardless of the references used. In addition, the prevalence of excess body weight, in overweight as well as in obesity, was significantly higher ($p<0.05$) in males in relation to females. Nevertheless, the percentage of overweight was significantly higher than obesity in both sexes when applying the international references.

Table 2 displays and compares the mean values of weight (kg), height (cm) and BMI (kg/m^2) corresponding to the different ages considered in the group of males who maintain normal nutrition at age 14 (standard group) or have excess weight (overweight and obesity groups). Mean values of registered weight were significantly higher ($p<0.05$) in every age considered in the groups with excess weight (overweight and obesity groups) with respect to the standard group, except for birth and age 1 year. There were not any statistically significant differences among mean values of height in the different groups at any considered age. Regarding BMI, the calculated mean values were significantly higher ($p<0.05$) in every age considered within the groups with excess body weight (overweight and obesity groups) with respect to the standard group, except for birth and age 1 year.

Table 1. Prevalence of excess body weight (overweight and obesity) at age 14 according to national and International references

	Ferrández et al.[17]		Cole et al.[18]	
	Males **n (%)**	**Females** **n (%)**	**Males** **n (%)**	**Females** **n (%)**
Overweight	55 (17.9%)	20 (6.7%)	76 (24.7%)	30 (10.1%)
Obesity	34 (11.1%)	18 (6.1%)	19 (6.2%)	11 (3.7%)
Total	89 (29.0%)	38 (12.8%)	95 (30.9%)	41 (13.8%)

Table 2. Mean values for weight, height and BMI in males

Weight (kg)			
Age (years)	Standard group M (SD)	Overweight group M (SD)	Obesity group M (DE)
0	3.32 (0.47)	3.39 (0.44)	3.32 (0.42)
1	10.14 (0.95)	10.28 (0.81)	10.66 (1.09)
2	12.84 (1.10)	13.31 (1.27)*	13.33 (1.56)*
3	15.12 (1.34)	15.85 (1.81)*	16.35 (1.96)*
4	17.42 (1.89)	18.31 (2.28)*	19.86 (2.23)*
6	21.82 (2.82)	24.31(3.44)*	26.82 (4.44)*
8	27.96 (4.15)	31.41 (4.01)*	37.14 (6.06)*
10	34.84 (5.38)	40.91 (4.68)*	47.92 (7.26)*
12	42.66 (6.56)	50.91 (8.27)*	63.81 (12.3)*
14	54.35 (8.16)	65.12 (8.30)*	81.47 (12.6)*
Height (cm)			
Age (years)	Standard group M (SD)	Overweight group M (SD)	Obesity group M (SD)
0	50.52 (2.20)	50.63 (2.02)	49.98 (2.26)
1	76.46 (2.66)	76.56 (1.93)	76.80 (2.53)
2	88.78 (2.89)	88.71 (3.06)	88.26 (3.02)
3	97.17 (2.88)	97.28 (2.81)	97.15 (3.45)
4	104.23 (3.86)	104.39 (3.91)	104.76 (4.11)
6	117.17 (4.60)	117.98 (4.24)	118.58 (4.53)
8	129.47 (5.29)	129.29 (4.80)	130.57 (5.21)
10	140.19 (5.80)	140.63 (5.30)	142.02 (6.61)
12	151.34 (7.49)	151.19 (7.78)	154.53 (7.30)
14	165.89 (8.19)	164.47 (8.33)	165.71 (7.17)
IMC (kg/m^2)			
Age (years)	Standard group M (SD)	Overweight group M (SD)	Obesity group M (SD)
0	12.98 (1.34)	13.22 (1.32)	12.92 (1.94)
1	17.35 (1.21)	17.48 (1.25)	18.02 (1.49)
2	16.29 (0.99)	16.80 (1.26)*	17.06 (1.23)*
3	16.07 (1.35)	16.72 (1.45)*	17.28 (1.47)*
4	15.94 (1.08)	16.76 (1.39)*	18.06 (1.27)*
6	15.92 (1.32)	17.42 (1.94)*	18.98 (2.26)*
8	16.62 (1.76)	18.67 (1.78)*	21.66 (2.40)*
10	17.68 (1.99)	20.63 (1.49)*	23.68 (2.56)*
12	18.55 (1.99)	21.90 (2.48)*	26.57 (3.60)*
14	19.67 (1.83)	23.80 (2.13)*	29.05 (4.74)*

(*) $p < 0.05$ with respect to standard group.

Table 3. Mean values for weight. height and BMI in females

Weight (kg)		
Age (years)	Standard group M (SD)	Overweight group M (SD)	Obesity group M (SD)
0	3.17 (0.40)	3.17 (0.38)	3.32 (0.52)
1	9.73 (1.26)	9.92 (1.28)	10.24 (1.08)
2	12.28 (1.33)	13.02 (1.51)*	14.60 (2.31)*
3	14.60 (1.56)	16.15 (2.05)*	18.65 (3.35)*
4	16.95 (2.18)	18.16 (2.56)*	21.62 (4.48)*
6	21.70 (3.03)	24.52 (3.51)*	28.95 (4.80)*
8	27.99 (4.18)	32.71 (4.96)*	41.50 (5.94)*
10	35.11 (6.11)	42.48 (6.18)*	51.68 (6.24)*
12	44.74 (7.47)	54.34 (10.1)*	65.50 (5.54)*
14	51.74 (6.67)	64.51 (6.61)*	77.12 (8.45)*
Height (cm)		
Age (years)	Standard group M (SD)	Overweight group M (SD)	Obesity group M (SD)
0	49.64 (2.07)	50.10 (2.06)	49.29 (2.31)
1	75.26 (2.66)	74.56 (2.61)	76.10 (2.68)
2	87.21 (3.00)	87.53 (3.26)	89.68 (4.06)*
3	96.59 (3.25)	97.88 (4.08)	98.97 (3.43)*
4	103.20 (3.87)	103.48 (4.63)	106.42 (4.68)*
6	116.66 (4.40)	118.18 (5.46)	119.12 (4.91)*
8	129.70 (5.09)	131.28 (5.55)	134.40 (4.53)*
10	140.16 (6.13)	142.67 (7.08)	144.73 (5.69)*
12	153.61 (7.05)	155.93 (8.23)	155.00 (5.72)
14	160.88 (5.94)	161.45 (6.37)	162.77 (4.97)
BMI (kg/m^2)		
Age (years)	Standard group M (SD)	Overweight group M (SD)	Obesity group M (SD)
0	12.84 (1.12)	12.64 (1.11)	13.60 (1.49)
1	17.10 (1.40)	17.64 (1.16)	17.66 (1.28)
2	16.14 (1.36)	17.01 (1.40)*	18.04 (1.81)*
3	15.95 (1.28)	16.83 (1.66)*	18.89 (2.25)*
4	15.87 (1.49)	16.89 (1.39)*	18.92 (2.71)*
6	15.89 (1.61)	17.47 (1.45)*	20.30 (2.26)*
8	16.93 (2.08)	18.92 (2.12)*	22.89 (2.26)*
10	17.69 (2.12)	20.79 (1.95)*	23.91 (2.90)*
12	18.71 (2.24)	22.21 (2.91)*	27.65 (1.27)*
14	19.95 (1.99)	24.22 (3.05)*	28.49 (3.64)*

(*) p<0.05 with respect to standard group.

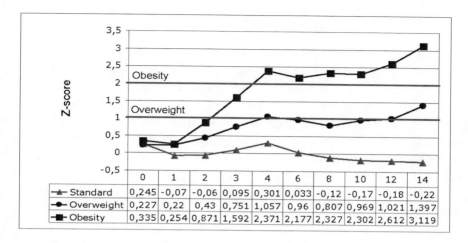

Figure 1. Evolution of mean values for BMI (Z-score).

Table 3 shows and analyzes mean values for weight (kg), height (cm) and BMI (kg/m^2) corresponding to every age considered in females who show normal nutrition status at age 14 years (standard group) or have excess body weight (overweight and obesity groups). Mean values of the registered weight were significantly higher ($p<0.05$) at every age considered within the groups with excess body weight (overweight and obesity) with respect to the standard group, but for birth and age 1 year. There were not any significant differences regarding mean values of registered height at any considered age among the normal and overweight groups; however, mean values of height were significantly higher ($p<0.05$) at 2, 3, 4, 6, 8 and 10 years of age within the obesity group with respect to the standard group. As for BMI, mean values were significantly higher ($p<0.05$) in every age considered within the groups with excess body weight (overweight and obesity groups) compared to the standard group, except for birth and age 1 year.

Figure 1 displays and compares mean values for BMI (Z-score) corresponding to the different ages of the groups whose individuals showed normal nutrition at age 14 (standard group) or have excess body weight (overweight and obesity group). Even when mean values for BMI (Z-score) were significantly higher ($p<0.05$) beyond 2 years of age within the groups with excess weight (overweight and obesity) with respect to the standard group, it was after 4 years of age when the values reached the range of overweight and obesity, respectively, and it would remain so until 14 years of age.

DISCUSSION

Excess body weight (overweight and obesity) is a multifactorial disorder whose pathogenesis includes genetic, metabolic, psychosocial and environmental factors. Nevertheless, this fast increase in its prevalence seems to be related to environmental factors, such as poor healthy nutrition habits and sedentary lifestyle (a decrease in physical activity in children and adolescents conditioned, to a great extent, by television and/or new technologies). It is precisely the *NAOS strategy* [14] that emerges as a response to that ascending trend to excess body weight in our society, pretending to promote a series of programs addressed to infant-juvenile population, whose dietary habits and lifestyle have not yet become established and are, therefore, improvable through education programs.

There are not uniform reference values, at present day, which allow a precise diagnosis of body mass index. Therefore, the epidemiological data that have been previously published with regard to this matter are quite variable and make international, and even national comparisons, fairly complicated [4, 19, 20]. However, the body mass index is considered an acceptable anthropometric parameter to define excess body weight [21, 24]. In this way, the application of international reference standards suggested by Cole et al. [18] is considered appropriate, although whenever there are local reference charts, their use is preferential. In this case, international as well as qualified national criteria have been applied to calculate the prevalence of excess body weight at age 14 years. The results we have obtained suggest, on one side, that one in every five adolescents present excess body weight at the end of the pediatric age, and it is basically similar regardless of the reference values applied; on the other side, they confirm that overweight and obesity affect males at a higher rate than women. Nevertheless, as it happened in this case, whenever the international standards from Cole et al. have been applied, the percentage of obesity show very low levels whereas overweight reaches relatively high levels. This means, it suggests that these reference values tend to underestimate obesity and overestimate overweight, which would justify the use of updated national references as more advisable in clinical practice, in the way we have done in this study.

The comparison of the rates of prevalence of excess body weight registered at age 14 with the results of different national and international studies that have been published applying the standards from Cole et al. reveals how the rate of prevalence of excess weight in our environment (one out of five adolescents at age 14) is basically similar to that of the rest of

Spanish regions [23, 25, 26] and geographic/cultural environment countries [4, 27-30]. However, we should remark how –in both sexes- adolescents who had excess body weight at age 14 years showed body mass index significantly higher at age 2 years with respect to those who presented with normal nutrition at age 14 and, in addition, these differences gradually increased throughout growing-up. This means, it seems that the excess body weight would be a nosological entity that begins at early stages in life in which diet depends almost exclusively on dietary habits and/or behavior in the familiar environment. It would later deteriorate at the time of school attendance, probably due to the acquisition of a certain degree of autonomy in feeding, since they usually do some of the daily intake out of their houses, in school lunch room or without family supervision. Finally, a disproportionate weight increase would take place during adolescence, especially in males, probably in relation to unhealthy acquired dietary habits and lifestyle.

The early onset of weight increase and its persistence throughout pediatric age, and consequently, the increase of risk of overweight/obesity in adult life, make the development of active policies in different areas of intervention mandatory: community and family, school, corporate and sanitary environments. On one side, families should get basic nutrition knowledge (institutional advertising, informational resources, interactive applications, etc.) in order to create healthy eating habits and/or lifestyles in children who, at the same time, would be given the education to develop them within school environment. Mass catering, and concretely school meals, is in an expansion stage as a consequence of new ways of social and familiar organization, and more and more every day, families delegate some of the meals of their children in these services and/or catering companies. School lunchroom is one of the most interesting instruments in school environment, since it could help strengthen acquired knowledge and healthy eating habits. This means, it would serve as a transmitter of nutrition education since the theoretical dietary proposals for quotidian life in adolescents would be adapted through it, so contributing to the affective adhesion to healthy dietary habits. We should remark that the deterioration of the dietary model is, to a great extent, conditioned by a high availability of food, and specifically, by a permissive accessibility to processed food (industrial pastries, soft drinks, sweets, chocolate, industrial fruit juices, etc.), whose consumption should be casual and means a higher calorie intake, as well as total fat and saturated fat, refined sugar and cholesterol. Considering school and familiar environment as the educational areas with the greatest influence for the acquisition of healthy eating habits and lifestyles, the attitude to be adopted by the school centers regarding nutrition aspects should be inherently exemplary in order to accomplish its educational purposes. Consequently, it would contribute to avoid infant-juvenile excess body weight (overweight and obesity). As an example, the limitation and/or modification of selling high calorie food in school centers (food and soft drinks vending machines) would be appropriate as a coherent pedagogic measure facing a health problem that is due to a lack of individual, familiar and social education. With regard to corporate area, food and beverage industry should commit in the development and commercial distribution of more healthy products by means of modifying the composition of food (low salt, saturated fat and refined sugar) and/or issuing nutrition information (food advertising, labeling, internet portals, etc.). Hospitality and restaurant services should offer varied and nutrition-balanced feeding that allowed the consumer to choose healthy options. Finally, with respect to sanitary environment, primary health care teams, and more specifically, pediatricians, should include a series of preventive measures to be applied within the preventive and health promotion programs in the first years of life, together with weight and height periodic control. Regular physical activity appropriate to every age should also be promoted, as well as the reinforcement of a series of general standards of behavior, such as respecting meal schedule, avoiding sedentary lifestyle and increase quotidian activity, reducing time for TV and/or new technologies, etc.

In order to achieve its goal (the promotion of healthy feeding and physical activity), the NAOS strategy proposed the creation of an Observatory of Obesity to assure a methodological homogeneity in the evaluation and monitoring of the different initiatives directed to get its main objectives. In this sense, the lack of a program for the prevention of child obesity in our community, which includes specialized attention with the aim to be the essential structure of the NAOS strategy, makes the patients with excess body weight depend on primary care pediatrician in our environment. Even when they do play an essential role in the early detection of excess body weight, they lack the necessary perspective a specialized consultation should have to interfere with the "natural evolution" of excess body weight, since it has more complete evidence-based information on epidemiological, clinical and evolution factors.

REFERENCES

[1]   Odgen CL, Flegal KM, Carroll MD, Johnson CL. Prevalence and trends in overweight among US children and adolescents, 1999-2000. JAMA 2002; 288:1728–32.

[2]   Tzotzas T, Krassas GE. Prevalence and trends of obesity in children and adults of South Europe. Pediatr Endocrinol Rev 2004; 1 (3 Suppl):448-54.

[3]   Schober E, Rami B, Kirchengast S, Waldhör T, Sefranek R. Recent trend in overweight and obesity in male adolescents in Austria: a population-based study. Eur J Pediatr 2007; 166:709–14.

[4]   Livingstone B. Epidemiology of childhood obesity in Europe. Eur J Pediatr 2000; 159 (1 Suppl):14–34.

[5]   Durá-Travé T, Hualde-Olascoaga J, Garralda-Torres I, Grupo Colaborador de Navarra. Overweight among children in Navarra (Spain) and its impact on adolescence. Med Clin (Barc) 2012; 138(2):52-6.

[6]   Reilly JJ, Armstrong J, Dorosty AR, Emmett PM, Ness A, Rogers I, Steer C, Sherriff A. Avon Longitudinal Study of Parents and Children Study Team. Early life risk factors for obesity in childhood: cohort study. BMJ 2005; 330 (7504):1357.

[7]   Johannsson E, Arngrimsson SA, Thorsdottir I, Sveinsson T. Tracking of overweight from early childhood to adolescence in cohorts born 1988 and 1994: overweight in a high birth weight population. Int J Obes (Lond) 2006; 30:1265–71.

[8]   Nader PR, O'Brien M, Houts R, Bradley R, Belsky J, Crosnoe R, Friedman S, Mei Z, Susman EJ. National Institute of Child Health and Human Development Early Child Care Research Network. Identifying risk for obesity in early childhood. Pediatrics 2006; 118 (3):e594-601.

[9]   Wright CM, Emmett PM, Ness AR, Reilly JJ, Sherriff, A. Tracking of obesity and body fatness through mid-childhood. Arch Dis Child 2010; 95:612–7.

[10]   Freedman DS, Khan LF, Serdula MK, Dietz WH, Srinivasan SR, Berenson GS. The relation of childhood BMI to adult adiposity: The Bogalusa Heart Study. Pediatrics 2005; 115:22–7.

[11]   Biro FM, Wien M. Childhood obesity and adult morbidities. Am J Clin Nutr 2010; 91:1499–505.

[12]   Field AE, Cook NR, Gillman MW. Weight status in childhood as a predictor of becoming overweight or hypertensive in early adulthood. Obes Res 2005; 13:163–9.

[13] Branca F, Nikogosian H, Lobstein T. The Challenge of Obesity in the WHO European Region and the Strategies for Response. World Health Organization. Copenhagen. 2007. Available at URL: http://www.euro.who.int/document/e89858.pdf

[14] Estrategia para la Nutrición, Actividad Física y Prevención de la Obesidad (NAOS). Ministerio de Sanidad, Servicios Sociales e Igualdad. Agencia Española de Seguridad Alimentaria y Nutrición (AESAN). Available at URL: http://www.naos.aesan.msssi.gob.es/ naos/ estrategia/ que_es/

[15] Durá-Travé T, Garralda-Torres I, Hualde-Olasgoaga J, Grupo Colaborador de Navarra. Longitudinal study of child growth in Navarre (1993-2007). *An Pediatr (Barc)* 2009; 70:526-33.

[16] Atención a la poblacion infantil y adolescente en Atención Primaria. Guía de actuación. Departamento de Salud. Gobierno de Navarra, Pamplona, 2000.

[17] Ferrández A, Baguer L, Labarta JL Labena C, Mayayo E, Puba B, et al. Longitudinal study of normal Spanish children from birth to adulthood (anthoprometric, pubertal, radiological and intellectual data. *Pediatr Endocr Rev* 2005; 2:423-559.

[18] Cole TJ, Bellizzi MC, Flegal KM, Dietz WH. Establishing a standard definition for child overweight and obesity worldwide: international survey. *BMJ* 2000; 320:1240-5.

[19] Serra L, Ribas L, Aranceta J, Pérez C, Saavedra P, Peña L. Childhood and adolescent obesity in Spain. Results of the enKid study (1998-2000). *Med Clin (Barc)* 2003; 21:725–32.

[20] Lobstein T, Frelut ML. Prevalence of overweight among children in Europe. *Obes Rev* 2003; 4:195–200.

[21] Dietz WH, Bellizzi M. Introduction: the use of body mass index to assess obesity in children. *Am J Clin Nutr* 1999; 70 (Suppl):123S–5S.

[22] Reilly JJ, Dorosty AR, Emmett PM. Identification of the obese child: adequacy of the body mass index for clinical practice and epidemiology. *Int J Obes* 2000; 24:1623–7.

[23] Marrodán MD, Mesa MS, Alba JA, Ambrosio B, Barrio PA, Drack L, et al. Obesity screening: updated criteria and their clinical and populational validity. *An Pediatr* (Barc) 2006; 65:5–14.

[24] Calañas-Continente A, Arrizabalaga JJ, Caixas A, Cordido F, Grupo de Trabajo sobre Obesidad (SEEN). Diagnostic and therapeutic recommendations for overweight and obesity during adolescence. *Med Clin* (Barc) 2010; 135:265–73.

[25] Larrañaga N, Amiano P, Arrizabalaga JJ, Bidaurrazaga J, Gorostiza E. Prevalence of obesity in 4-18-year-old population in the *Basque Country, Spain. Obes Rev* 2007; 8:281–7.

[26] Martínez V, Sánchez M, Moya P, Solera M, Notario B, Salcedo F, et al. Trends in excess weight and thinness among Spanish schoolchildren in the period 1992-2004: the Cuenca study. *Public Health Nutr* 2009; 12:1015–8

[27] Krassas GE, Tzotzas T, Tsametis C, Konstantinidis T. Prevalence and trends in overweight and obesity among children and adolescents in Thessaloniki, Greece. *J Pediatr Endocrinol Metab* 2001; 14 (5 Suppl):1319–26.

[28] Wang Y, Monteiro C, Popkin BM. Trends of obesity and underweight in older children and adolescents in the United States, Brazil, China, and Russia. *Am J Clin Nutr* 2002; 75:971–7.

[29] Lissau I, Overpeck MD, Ruan WJ, Due P, Holstein BE, Hediger ML. Health Behaviour in School-aged Children Obesity Working Group. Body mass index and overweight in adolescents in 13 European countries, Israel, and the United States. *Arch Pediatr Adolesc Med* 2004; 158:27-33.

[30] Zimmermann MB, Gübeli C, Püntener C, Molinari L. Detection of overweight and obesity in a national sample of 6-12-y-old Swiss children: accuracy and validity of reference values for body mass index from the US Centers for Disease Control and Prevention and the International Obesity Task Force. *Am J Clin Nutr* 2004; 79:838–43.

In: Focus on Nutrition …
Editor: Teodoro Durá-Travé

ISBN: 978-1-63463-223-2
© 2015 Nova Science Publishers, Inc.

Chapter 4

DIETARY PATTERNS IN CHILDREN WITH ATTENTION DEFICIT HYPERACTIVITY DISORDER TREATED WITH EXTENDED-RELEASE METHYLPHENIDATE

Teodoro Durá-Travé[1,2], Fidel Gallinas-Victoriano[2],
Sada Elena Zarikian-Denis[2], Aida González-Benavides[2]
and María Garcia-Ayerra[2]
[1] Department of Pediatrics, Faculty of Medicine,
University of Navarra, Pamplona, Spain
[2] Department of Pediatrics, Navarra Hospital Complex, Pamplona, Spain

ABSTRACT

Objective: To assess the feeding pattern in a group of patients previously diagnosed with attention deficit hyperactivity disorder (ADHD) and under treatment with extended-release methylphenidate (MPH-ER).

Material and methods: A nutrition survey (food intake recall for three consecutive days) was conducted in a sample of 100 patients diagnosed with ADHD in treatment with MPH-ER, and 100 healthy children (control group). The intake of calories and nutrients, as well as the nutrition status, were monitored and subsequently compared in both groups.

Results: Nutritional status in ADHD group was significantly lower (p<0.05) than in control group. Calorie intake in mid-morning snack, lunch and afternoon snack was significantly higher (p<0.05) in the control group. Calorie intake in dinner was significantly higher (p<0.05) in the ADHD group. No significant differences were found in breakfast. Total calorie intake, as well as the intake of proteins, carbohydrates, fat, fiber, calcium, iron, magnesium, zinc, selenium and phosphorous, thiamine, niacin, vitamin B6 and folate in control group was significantly higher than in ADHD group.

Conclusions: The daily intake of calories and nutrients in patients diagnosed with ADHD under treatment with MPH-ER is, generally, lower than in healthy population of similar age. Consideration should be given to the need to share programs of nutrition education simultaneously with multimodal treatment so as to avoid the nutrition consequences of treatment with MPH.

INTRODUCTION

Multimodal treatment in Attention Deficit Hyperactivity disorder (ADHD) is a combination of psychosocial intervention with drug therapy, which usually implies prolonged therapy with a long-acting stimulant medication [1-4]. Stimulant drugs, and specifically methylphenidate (MPH), are first-line treatment in patients diagnosed with ADHD. Many clinical trials confirm the sustained efficacy of MPH in attentional and behavioral symptoms, that allows, in most cases, the optimization of the child's academic, familiar and social situation [2, 3, 5-9].

In Spain, there are two preparations of extended-release methylphenidate (MPH-ER): one is an osmotic-controlled release oral delivery system (OROS-MPH) and the other one consists of double action microspheres or modified-release methylphenidate (MR-MPH) [10]. The pharmacokinetic properties of these prolonged release formulations guarantee relatively constant plasma levels in the course of the day in contrast to immediate release formulations [11]. This fact could hypothetically affect appetite in different meals along the day owing to the hyporexia that is associated to the administration of methylphenidate.

In fact, the nutritional status in patients with ADHD tends to worsen in prolonged treatment with MPH-ER [12, 13], and justifies the interest to know the dietary intake of these patients throughout the treatment. The purpose of this chapter is to monitor the caloric and nutrients intake dietary patterns in a group of patients diagnosed with ADHD under treatment with MPH-ER, and to analyze the need to design nutrition intervention strategies in these patients.

MATERIAL AND METHODS

Patients

A nutrition survey has been conducted in the first 100 patients diagnosed with ADHD in the neuropediatric unit of the "Complejo Hospitalario de Navarra" who attended follow-up consultation within the year 2012 (the nutrition survey was carried out between January and April).

All patients should be under exclusive and maintained treatment with OROS-MPH or MR-MPH for at least 12 months. The criteria from the last edition of the *Diagnostic and Statistical Manual of Mental Disorders* (DSM-IV-R) were applied for diagnosis and classification [14]. Patients were grouped in two clinical subtypes: those who showed mainly attention deficit of *inattentive subtype* and those who presented attention deficit, hyperactivity and impulsivity or *combined subtype*. Another nutrition survey was carried out simultaneously in 100 healthy patients (50 males and 50 females) of similar ages.

Patients and/or controls who suffered from any known chronic disease which could condition the nutrition status and those who took any energy, mineral of vitamin supplements were also excluded.

Nutrition Survey

The nutrition survey was conducted as a personal interview at the time of consultation using a food intake registration of three consecutive school days. Every patient was asked about food intake in every meal during the previous three consecutive days (breakfast, mid-morning snack, lunch, afternoon snack and dinner). A photograph album with portions and measures from the *Institut Scientifique et Technique de la Nutrition et de l´Alimentation* (París, 2002) [15] was used to calculate the size of the corresponding portions of the different foods.

The intake of calories and nutrients (proteins, carbohydrates, total fat, saturated fatty acid –SFA-, monounsaturated fatty acids –MUFA- and polyunsaturated fatty acids –PUFA-, total fiber and cholesterol), minerals (calcium, iron, iodine, magnesium, zinc, selenium, and phosphorus), and vitamins (thiamine, riboflavin, niacin, vitamin B6, folate, vitamin B12, vitamin C, vitamin A, vitamin D and vitamin E) was calculated using the CESNID 1.0® nutrition calculation software (Centro de Enseñanza Superior de Nutrición y Dietética. Universidad de Barcelona) [16].

Nutrition Study

Sex, age, clinical subtype and MPH dose (mg/kg/day), weight, height, triceps skinfold and mid-upper arm circumference from every patient and control were recorded. Weight and height assessment were done in underclothes and barefoot. Weight was measured using an Año-Sayol® scale (read range 0-120 kg and precision 100 g) and height was measured using a wall mounted rigid stadiometer (ranking 60-210 cm and with 0.1 cm precision). A constant pressure Holtain-type skinfold calliper was used to measure triceps skinfold. Weight, height and mid-upper arm circumference Z-scores as well as body mass index (BMI) were calculated using the SEINAPTRACKER program (Medicalsoft Intercath, S.L. Universidad de Barcelona, 2007-2008). Reference growth curves and charts were the Centro Andrea Prader (Zaragoza, 2002) charts.

Results are displayed as means (M) with standard deviation (SD). Statistical analysis was done using the *IMB SPSS Statistics program 20 version* (Chicago, Illinois, EE.UU.). Statistical significance was reported when $p < 0.05$.

RESULTS

The sample of patients consisted in 68 males and 32 females, with a male/female ratio of 2.1. Combined subtype represented 61% of cases and inattentive subtype accounted for 39%. The proportion of combined subtype was significantly higher ($p < 0.001$) in males (67.6%) than in females (46.8%). Mean age of patients was 11.4 years (CI 95%: 11.13-11.67) and there were not any statistically significant differences in comparison with the control group (mean age: 11.2 years, CI 95%: 10.91-11.49).

All patients surveyed were under treatment with MPH-ER for a mean time of 27.9 months (CI 95%: 24.8-31.1) and a mean dose of 1.01 mg/kg/day (CI 95%: 0.96-1.06). Sixty-three patients were treated with OROS-MPH at a mean dose of 1.07 mg/kg/day (CI 95%: 0.99-1.15) and thirty seven were treated with MR-MPH at a mean dose of 0.90 mg/kg/day (CI 95%: 0.81-0.99), being this difference not significant.

Table 1 shows and compares the results of the nutrition study in both groups. The mean values of weight (Z-score), height (Z-score), BMI (Z-score), mid-upper arm circumference (Z-score) and triceps skinfold (cm) in the ADHD group were significantly lower than in control group.

Table 1. Results of the nutrition study in both groups

Item	ADHD Group M (DS)	Control Group M (DS)	p
Weight (Z score)	-0.729 (0.88)	-0.196 (1.10)	<0.001
Height (Z score)	-0.219 (0.99)	+0.095 (1.10)	<0.040
BMI (Z score)	-0.805 (0.77)	-0.360 (0.97)	<0.001
MUAC (Z score)	-0.578 (0.89)	-0.084 (1.07)	<0.001
TS (cm)	12.7 (5.2)	16.3 (6.8)	<0.001

MUAC: mid-upper arm circumference. TS: triceps skinfold.

Table 2 displays and compares the total daily and every meal calorie intake (breakfast, mid-morning snack, lunch, afternoon snack and dinner) in both groups.

Total daily calorie intake, as well as mid-morning snack, lunch and afternoon snack energy intake were significantly higher (p< 0.05) in control group with respect to ADHD group. In contrast, dinner calorie intake was significantly higher (p<0.05) in ADHD group than in control group. No significant differences were found in breakfast energy intake between both groups.

Furthermore, there were not any significant differences among total daily calorie intake and each daily meal (breakfast, mid-morning snack, lunch, afternoon snack and dinner) in patients treated with OROS-MPH or MR-MPH.

Table 3 sets out and compares the daily intake of macronutrients, minerals and vitamins for both groups. Within the control group, the daily intake of some macronutrients (proteins, carbohydrates, total fat, MUFA, PUFA and total fiber), minerals (calcium, iron, magnesium, zinc, selenium and phosphorus) and vitamins (thiamine, niacin, vitamin B6 and folate) was significantly higher (p<0.05) than in ADHD group. In control group, the Recommended Daily Intake (RDIs) for minerals and vitamins was sufficiently fulfilled except for calcium, iodine, vitamin A, vitamin D and vitamin E. In contrast, in ADHD group, the RDIs corresponding to calcium, iodine, magnesium, folate, vitamin A, vitamin D and vitamin E were not adequately covered.

Table 2. Total daily calorie intake and from different meals in both groups

Intake	ADHD Group M (DS)	Control Group M (DS)	p
Breakfast	322.4 (137.4)	313.8 (94.7)	<0.616
Mid-morning snack	148.2 (128.2)	263.2 (105.4)	<0.001
Lunch	401.5 (176.1)	735.3 (175.7)	<0.001
Mid-afternoon snack	267.6 (136.6)	312.4 (102.3)	<0.011
Dinner	577.0 (205.3)	477.6 (169.0)	<0.001
TOTAL	1.786.5 (335.9)	2.061.1 (242.4)	<0.001

Table 3. Daily intake of macronutrients, minerals and vitamins in both groups

Nutrients	ADHD group M (DS)	Control group M (DS)	p
Proteins (g)	82.2 (19.3)	98.6 (20.0)	<0.001
Carbohydrates (g)	207.0 (54.2)	250.9 (45.0)	<0.001
Total fat(g)	63.4 (19.2)	69.4 (18.6)	<0.028
SFA (g)	26.72 (8.5)	28.6 (8.2)	<0.122
MUFA (g)	22.5 (7.8)	24.8 (7.9)	<0.047
PUFA(g)	7.2 (2.5)	8.7 (2.6)	<0.001
Total fiber (g)	15.1 (6.3)	23.8 (12.2)	<0.001
Cholesterol (mg)	313.7 (127.7)	302.9 (103.2)	<0.522
Calcium (mg)	787.8 (201.5)	877.0 (204.7)	<0.003
Iron (mg)	13.5 (5.0)	17.1 (5.8)	<0.001
Iodine (µg)	76.6 (22.6)	80.0 (20.3)	<0.266
Magnesium (mg)	223.1 (51.5)	295.2 (88.9)	<0.001
Zinc (mg)	8.7 (2.5)	10.2 (2.7)	<0.001
Selenium (µg)	111.8 (54.3)	133.3 (42.8)	<0.001
Phosphorous (mg)	1.344.3 (305.0)	1.550.1 (305.7)	<0.001
Thiamine (mg)	1.5 (0.5)	1.7 (0.5)	<0.019
Riboflavin (mg)	1.8 (0.5)	1.9 (0.5)	<0.528
Niacin (mg)	33.7 (9.1)	38.2 (8.7)	<0.001
Vitamin B_6(mg)	1.7 (0.6)	2.0 (0.7)	<0.001
Folate (µg)	220.8 (109.2)	301.6 (151.5)	<0.001
Vitamin B_{12}(mg)	5.9 (3.9)	5.5 (3.3)	<0.451
Vitamin C (mg)	48.0 (34.7)	58.4 (36.6)	<0.460

Nutrients	ADHD group M (DS)	Control group M (DS)	p
Vitamin A (µg)	486.0 (312.2)	438.9 (204.0)	<0.223
Vitamin D (µg)	4.3 (2.8)	4.1 (2.8)	<0.744
Vitamin E (mg)	5.4 (1.6)	5.8 (1.6)	<0.120

DISCUSSION

Among the epidemiological aspects of this series, it is remarkable the presence of a slight male predominance (male/female ratio: 2.1) and the higher prevalence of the combined subtype. This aspects match with the references [17, 18]. This fact makes us consider this sample as representative of an average population of patients diagnosed with ADHD and, as a consequence, no statistical bias in results or conclusions in this sense was suspected.

The condition for inclusion in this chapter was a long-time and exclusive therapy with MPH-ER: OROS-MPH or MR-MPH, since the pharmacokinetic properties result in a better compliance and make them preferable to other immediate release formulations [9, 11, 19, 20]. In any case, the time of administration should be personalized, given the interindividual variability in plasma concentrations and/or the duration of therapeutic effect. It should be adapted to schedule, academic and behavioural needs, which requires an adjustment of dosage in relation to the clinical response. In this series, dosage of MPH was within safety and tolerability margins, since in any case was the prescribed dose manifestly high (maximum dose as 1.68 mg/kg/day) to lead to the possibility of suspending treatment in order to avoid secondary effects [2, 7, 21-23].

Pharmaceutical preparations of immediate release methylphenidate start clinical action 20 minutes after administration and get maximum plasma concentrations one hour after administration; the therapeutic effects last for approximately 4-5 hours. However, each OROS-MPH tablet has 22% MPH in its cover which releases immediately, and the remaining 78% releases slowly through an osmotic controlled-release mechanism. By doing so, a high plasma concentration is rapidly obtained (in 1-2 hours), followed by an ascending prolonged release with a maximum plasma concentration in 6-7 hours and a duration of action of 10-12 hours. The MR-MPH tablets have 50% of microspheres that are covered by an antacid substance that prevents the dilution in stomach and therefore present extended release and/or action. The remaining 50% are non-covered microspheres and have immediate absorption and/or release. Therefore, the pharmacokinetic profile implies a more intense immediate action and a lesser extended action with respect to OROS-MPH, being its duration of action of approximately 7-8 hours [10].

However, it should be considered that searching and finding a sustained therapeutic effect during the day with the different MPH-ER preparations might also lead to an increase and/or lengthening of the secondary effects such as appetite loss in those meals whose period of time coincide with ascending plasma concentrations of MPH. In normal conditions, the administration of MPH-ER usually coincides with breakfast –between 8:00 and 9:00 AM- in order to adjust its predictable therapeutic effect to the academic and/or social schedule of the patient. However, this circumstance inevitably entails the coincidence of ascending or maximum concentration and the time for mid-morning snack and lunch, and so this chronological overlap could interfere in the nutritional optimization of these patients.

The results obtained in this survey highlight how treatment with MPH-ER modifies substantially the percent distribution of calorie intake of the different meals, most likely in relation to the pharmacokinetic curves. In fact, those patients diagnosed with ADHD under continued therapy with OROS-MPH or MR-MPH present a significant reduction of calorie intake in mid-morning snack as well as in lunch, and even extended until afternoon snack. This fact would be explained by the overlap of the time of the different meals and the maximum plasma concentrations of the components of immediate and extended release of these formulations, respectively. Subsequently, and after the therapeutic effect has presumably ended, a rebound effect was manifested as an relatively exaggerated increase in appetite at the time of dinner, which, consequently, would explain the higher calorie intake of these patients compared to the control group. However, this "bulimia-like" effect was not intense enough to make calorie and nutrients intake (macronutrients, minerals and vitamins) similar to healthy population of the same age. This means, patients under treatment with OROS-MPH or MR-MPH eat breakfast as children of the same age do, but simultaneously with the beginning of the pretended therapeutic effects, a loss of appetite manifests specially during breakfast and lunch time and, to a lesser extent, mid-afternoon snack. A rebound effect appears at dinner time, but this effect is not enough to compensate the lower calorie and nutrients intake consequence of the lower consumption of food throughout the day. This eventuality could be counterproductive in these patients since a continuous lower calorie and nutrients intake could affect the cognitive functions and, therefore, worsen the school abilities [24-26].

Even though daily mean intake of macronutrients (proteins, carbohydrates, fat, total fiber) as well as some minerals (calcium, iron, magnesium, zinc, selenium, phosphate) and vitamins (thiamine, niacin, vitamin B6, folate) was significantly higher in control group than in ADHD group, the recommended dietary intake for minerals and vitamins was virtually covered in both groups. This fact would explain that these patients do not develop specific nutrient deficiencies every so often despite a lower nutrition status [12, 27-30].

This chapter has methodological limitations. A group of ADHD in the absence of methylphenidate treatment has not been included because of ethical implications. Therefore, the results of caloric and nutrient intake and nutritional status of the patients have been compared with those from a group of healthy children of similar ages. Setting up a control group of patients with mild to moderate ADHD who were receiving no pharmacological treatment proved to be impracticable. The total number of patients in these circumstances who were followed was rather limited. Many of them finally required methylphenidate due to progressive psychosocial and/or educational deterioration, and the rest faced diagnostic uncertainty.

In conclusion, daily calorie and nutrient intake in patients under continuous treatment with MPH-ER are, in general, slightly lower than healthy people of the same age. This would justify the fact that the nutritional parameters registered in these patients were also significantly lower. Therefore, the need to dispense programs of nutritional education to the patients and/or their families simultaneously with multimodal treatment should be considered.

In addition, the application of nutrition strategies, such as increasing calorie intake by offering "favourite" foods and/or adding energy supplements, especially in mid-morning snack and lunch, could avoid the nutritional consequences of the treatment with MPH-ER.

REFERENCES

[1]   American Academy of Child and Adolescent Psychiatry. Practice parameter for the use of stimulant medications in the treatment of children, adolescents, and adults. *J Am Acad Child Adolesc Psychiatry* 2002; 41(suppl 2):26-49.

[2]   Wilens T, McBurnett K, Stein M, Lerner M, Spencer T, Wolraich M. ADHD treatment with once-daily OROS methylphenidate: final results

from a long-term open-label study. J Am Acad Child Adolesc Psychiatry 2005; 44:1015-1023.

[3]   Brown RT, Amler RW, Freeman WS, et al. American Academy of Pediatrics, Committee on Quality Improvement, Subcommittee on Attention-Deficit/Hyperactivity Disorder. Treatment of attention-deficit/hyperactivity disorder: overview of the evidence. *Pediatrics* 2005; 115:e749-e757.

[4]   Molina BS, Hinshaw SP, Swanson JM, et al. MTA Cooperative Group. The MTA at 8 years: prospective follow-up of children treated for combined-type ADHD in a multisite study. *J Am Acad Child Adolesc Psychiatry* 2009; 48:484-500.

[5]   American Academy of Pediatrics. Clinical practice guideline: diagnosis and evaluation of the child with attention-deficit/hyperactivity disorder. *Pediatrics* 2000; 105:1158-1170.

[6]   Swanson J, Gupta S, Williams L, et al. Efficacy of a new pattern of delivery of methylphenidate for the treatment of ADHD: effects on activity level in the classroom and on the playground. *J Am Acad Child Adolesc Psychiatry* 2002; 41:1306-1314.

[7]   Kutcher S, Aman M, Brooks SJ, et al. International consensus statement on attention-deficit/hyperactivity disorder (ADHD) and disruptive behaviour disorders (DBDs): clinical implications and treatment practice suggestions. *European Neuropsychopharmacology* 2004; 14:11-28.

[8]   Rappley MD. Attention deficit-hyperactivity disorder. *N Engl J Med* 2005; 352:165-173.

[9]   National Institute for Health and Clinical Excellence (NICE). Attention-deficit/hyperactivity disorder (ADHD). London, UK. 2009. Available at URL: http://www.nice.org.uk/nicemedia/pdf/ADHDFullGuideline.pdf

[10]   Spanish Agency for Medicines and Health Products. Ministry of Health, Social Services and Equality. Available at URL: http://www.aemps.gob.es/cima/fichasTecnicas.do?metodo=buscar

[11]   Montañés-Rada F, Gangoso-Fermoso AB, Martínez-Granero MA. Drugs for attention deficit hyperactivity disorder. *Rev Neurol* 2009; 48:469-481.

[12]   Durá-Travé T, Yoldi-Petri ME, Zardoya-Santos P. Nutrition and attention deficit hyperactivity disorder: developmental follow-up of the anthropometric variables of a group of patients receiving treatment with osmotic controlled-release methylphenidate. *Rev Neurol* 2011; 53:257-264.

[13] Durá-Travé T, Yoldi-Petri ME, Gallinas-Victoriano F, Zardoya-Santos P. Effects of osmotic-release methylphenidate on height and weight in children with attention-deficit hyperactivity disorder (ADHD) following up to four years of treatment. *J Child Neurol* 2012; 27:604-609.

[14] American Psychiatric Association. In: *Diagnostic and Statistical Manual of Mental Disorders. 4th ed.* Washington, DC: American Psychological Association. 2000.

[15] SU.VI.MAX. Portions Alimentaires. Manuel photos pour l'estimation des quantités. Ed. *Polytechnica.* Paris. 2002.

[16] *Centre d'Ensenyament Superior de Nutrició i Dietètica.* Programa de cálculo nutricional CESNID 1.0 (Cd-rom). Universitat de Barcelona: *McGraw-Hill.* 2003.

[17] Cardo E, Severa-Barceló M. The prevalence of attention deficit hyperactivity disorder. *Rev Neurol* 2005; 40 (suppl 1):S11-S15.

[18] Froelich TE, Lanphear BP, Epstein JN, Barbaresi WJ, Katusic SK, Kahn RS. Prevalence, recognition, and treatment of attention-deficit/hyperactivity disorder in a national sample of US children. *Arch Pediatr Adolesc Med* 2007; 161: 857-864

[19] Banaschewski T, Coghill D, Santosh P, et al. Long-acting medications for the hyperkinetic disorders. *Eur Child Adolesc Psychiatry* 2006; 15: 476-495.

[20] Faraone SV, Biederman J, Spencer T, Aleardi M. Comparing the efficacy of medications for ADHD using meta-analysis. *Med Gen Med* 2006; 8: 4.

[21] MTA Cooperative Group. National Institute of Mental Health. Multimodal treatment Study of ADHD Follow-up. Changes in effectiveness and growth after the end of treatment. *Pediatrics* 2008; 113: 762-769.

[22] Charach A, Figueroa M, Chen S, Ickowics A, Schachar R. Stimulant treatment over 5 years: effects on growth. *J Am Acad Child Adolesc Psychiatry* 2006; 45:415-421.

[23] Wilens TE, McBurnett K, Bukstein O, et al. Multisite controlled study of OROS methylphenidate in the treatment of adolescents with attention-deficit/hyperactivity disorder. *Arch Pediatr Adolesc Med* 2006; 160:82-90.

[24] Stebenson J. Dietary influences on cognitive development and behaviour in children. *Proc Nutr Soc* 2006; 65:361-365.

[25] Bellisle F. Effects of diet on behaviour and cognition in children. Br J Nutr 2004; 92 (Suppl 2): 227-232.

[26]   Kar BR, Rao SL, Chandramouli BA. Cognitive development in children with chronic protein energy malnutrition. *Behav Brain Funct* 2008; 4: 31-33.

[27]   Arnold LE, Bozzolo H, Hollway J, et al. Serum zinc correlates with parent- and teacher-rated inattention in children with attention-deficit/hyperactivity disorder. *J Child Adolesc Psychopharmacol* 2005; 15: 628–636.

[28]   Quintero J, Rodríguez-Quirós J, Correas-Lauffer J, Pérez-Templado J. Nutritional aspects of attention-deficit/hyperactive disorder. *Rev Neurol* 2009; 49: 307-312.

[29]   Kiddie JY, Weiss MD, Kitts DD, Levy-Milne R, Wasdell MB. Nutritional status of children with attention deficit hyperactivity disorder: a pilot study. *Int J Pediatr* 2010; doi: 2010:767318.

[30]   Menegassi M, Mello ED, Guimarães LR, et al. Food intake and serum levels of iron in children and adolescents with attention-deficit/hyperactivity disorder. *Rev Bras Psiquiatr* 2010; 32:132-138.

In: Focus on Nutrition …
Editor: Teodoro Durá-Travé

ISBN: 978-1-63463-223-2
© 2015 Nova Science Publishers, Inc.

Chapter 5

DIETARY PATTERN IN SCHOOLCHILDREN WITH NORMAL NUTRITIONAL STATUS IN NAVARRE, SPAIN

Beatriz Durá-Gúrpide[1], Teodoro Durá-Travé[1,2], Fidel Gallinas-Victoriano[2], Marta Martínez-Merino[2] and Abel Justo-Ranera[2]

[1] Department of Pediatrics, Faculty of Medicine, University of Navarra, Pamplona, Spain
[2] Department of Pediatrics, Navarra Hospital Complex, Pamplona, Spain

ABSTRACT

Objective: To perform a nutritional assessment of the dietary model in a group of primary school students (9-12 years) with a normal nutritional status.

Material and methods: Food consumption was recorded over three consecutive school days in a sample of 353 primary school students (188 boys and 165 girls) with normal nutritional situations. The intake of energy, macronutrients, minerals, and vitamins was calculated and compared with the recommended intakes.

Results: The mean value of daily calorie intake was 2066.9 kcal. Cereals (33%), dairy products (19%), and meats (17%) represented 70% of the total caloric intake. Proteins contributed 20.3% of the calorie intake, sugars made up another 48.8%, total fat was 30.9%, and saturated fats composed 12.6%. Cholesterol intake was judged as excessive and 2/3 of the caloric intake was of animal origin. The mean intakes of calcium, iodine and A, D, and E vitamins were lower than the recommended dietary intakes.

Conclusions: The dietary model of primary school students with normal nutritional statuses varies from the Mediterranean prototype, characterized by an excessive intake of meats, a limited intake of cereals and dairy products, and a deficient intake of vegetables, fruits, legumes, and fish. This leads to an increase in the intake of proteins and fats from animals, which is detrimental to complex carbohydrate consumption and results in a deficient intake of calcium, iodine, and vitamins A, D, and E.

INTRODUCTION

Dietary habits have always been a social and cultural referent of different societies. However, scientific evidence in recent years has been essential in the consideration of dietary habits of a concrete population as a social and sanitary indicator [1]. The nutritional habits traditionally observed in some countries of the Mediterranean area have created the concept of a "Mediterranean diet", whose nutritional interest is based in the variety of foods included in it. In fact, every food group is allowed in adequate proportions and a balanced calorie and nutrient intake is guaranteed by means of a combination of fruits and vegetables with bread, pasta, and rice, legumes, dairy products, fish, and red meat, in addition to olive oil being used a cooking fat [2-4].

Nevertheless, the industrialization and increasing production of processed food are leading to a series of changes in eating habits and preferences in wide sectors of the population. Occidental society has accepted a dietary pattern characterized by an excessive intake of food from animal origins, especially meat and derivatives, as well as added sugars, at the expense of the intake of cereals, vegetables, and fruits. This fact is leading to an increase of saturated fat and cholesterol in the diet of many populations [5-8]. This deterioration of dietary patterns in our social and cultural environment is creating a concern about the gradual disappearance of the Mediterranean diet [9, 10]. This concern is the reason that justifies, to a great extent, studying the quality of feeding habits in the general population with special care for the sectors of the population who are more susceptible to influence, such as the infant population. On the other side, we assume that schoolchildren with normal nutritional statuses have eating habits that guarantee the necessary energy and nutrient requirements – without deficiencies or excess – and that those habits would contribute to the prevention of adult diseases, such as ischemic coronary disease, atherosclerosis, osteoporosis, obesity, diabetes, and high blood pressure, etc. [11-19].

The aim of this chapter is to achieve a descriptive study of eating habits in a group of primary education students with normal nutritional statuses. Also, we are attempting to analyze the adequacy of energy and nutrient intake in these schoolchildren in relation to the established nutritional requirements in order to design nutritional intervention strategies.

MATERIAL AND METHODS

Patients

A nutritional survey was conducted in a randomly selected group of 353 students (188 males and 165 females) in primary education (3rd to 6th grade: 9-12 years old) in the city of Pamplona in 2014 (the nutritional survey was carried out between January and June). All of those schoolchildren who suffered from any acute or chronic disease that might condition their nutritional status, those who use energy and/or vitamin and mineral supplements, and all those students who had lunch from their own home (from the home of relatives, school lunch, etc.) were excluded. The normality of the nutritional status was the condition sine qua non to be included in this study; this means that BMI should range between a standard deviation of +1 and -1 (Z-score).

Nutritional Survey

The nutritional survey was carried out in the form of personal interviews using a food intake registration for three consecutive school days. Every patient was asked about food intake in every meal during the previous three consecutive days (breakfast, mid-morning snack, lunch, afternoon snack and dinner). A photo album with portions and measures from the *Institut Scientifique et Technique de la Nutrition et de l´Alimentation* (Paris, 2002) [20] was used to calculate the size of the corresponding portions of the different foods that the participants reported to have eaten.

The foods were divided into the following groups:

1) Milk and dairy products
2) Cereals and cereal products
3) Sweets, bakery products, and pastry
4) Fruits and natural juices
5) Fats and oils
6) Meat and derivatives
7) Eggs and derivatives
8) Vegetables and tubers
9) Legumes
10) Fishes

Energy and nutrient consumption (proteins, carbohydrates, total fat, SFA, MUFA and PUFA, total fiber, and cholesterol), minerals (calcium, iron, iodine, magnesium, zinc, selenium, and phosphorus), and vitamins (thiamine, riboflavin, niacin, vitamin B6, folate, vitamin B12, vitamin C, vitamin A, vitamin D, and vitamin E) were calculated using the CESNID 1.0® nutritional calculation program (Centro de Enseñanza Superior de Nutrición y Dietética. Universidad de Barcelona [21]. The reference values for mineral and vitamin dietary reference intakes (DRIs) for different ages are from the updated tables of the National Academy of Sciences [22].

Nutritional Study

The sex, age, weight, and height of all the schoolchildren were recorded. Weight and height assessments were done in underclothes and in bare feet. Weight was measured using an Año-Sayol® scale (read range 0-120 kg and precision 100 g) and height was measured using a wall-mounted rigid stadiometer (ranking 60-210 cm and with 0.1 cm precision). BMI Z-scores were calculated using the SEINAPTRACKER program (Medicalsoft Intercath, S.L. Universidad de Barcelona, 2007-2008). Reference growth curves and charts were the Centro Andrea Prader (Zaragoza, 2004) charts.

Results are shown as means (M) and percentages (%) with corresponding standard deviations (SD) of confidence intervals (95% CI). The SPSS version 20.0 (Chicago, Illinois, USA) program was used for statistics and analysis (Student's T test, comparisons of proportions). Statistical significance was assumed for any p value<0.05.

Note: As there were no statistically significant differences in results among gender, they are shown together (consumption frequencies, nutrient and calorie intake, and percentage contribution of food groups)

RESULTS

Characteristics of the Sample

The average age of the surveyed students was 10.5 (CI 95%: 10.3-11.7), and there were no statistically significant differences between the two sexes. In the same way, there were no significant differences in the mean values for weight (males: 38.8±0.8 and females: 39.0±0.7), height (males: 143±0.6 and females: 142.8±0.7), and BMI (males: 18.6±0.1 and females: 18.42±0.3). All of the survey respondents described having lunch and dinner; however, 1.1% (n=4), 5.9% (n=21), and 3.1% (n=11) reported not having breakfast, lunch, or an afternoon snack, respectively.

Consumption Frequencies

Dairy products (91.5%), sweets, bakery products, and pastries (50%), and/or cereals (43%) and, to a lesser extent, fruits and natural juices (14%) and fats and oils (12%) were the food groups with high consumption as a form of breakfast. In addition, 72% and 15% of the respondents reported the addition of cocoa powder and sugar to milk, respectively. A glass of milk was the only intake for breakfast for 14% of the respondents.

As for the mid-morning snack, bread (61%), together with cured meat (46%), fruits (12%), and yogurt (11%) were the most frequently consumed foods.

In terms of lunch, meat (74%), as well as cereals (67%), dairy products (45%), fruits (37%), legumes (30%), vegetables (26%), tubers (18%), and fish (15%) were the most frequently consumed foods. 52% of the surveyed students reported the consumption of bread for lunch and 13% also consumed fried potatoes as a garnish for their meat or fish.

For the mid-afternoon snack, bread (78.2%), along with cured meat (42%), chocolate, and/or cocoa butter (26%), and, to a lesser extent, yogurt (13%) and fruits (8%), were the foods with the highest consumption rates.

Dairy products (77%), meats (69%), cereals (60%), vegetables (24%), tubers (20%), eggs (19%), fruits (19%), and fish (15%) were the foods with the highest consumption rate at dinner. Additionally, 53% of the surveyed students said that they regularly consume bread for dinner.

Nutrient and Calorie Intake

The average value of daily calorie intake was 2066.9 Kcal (CI 95%: 2040.2-2093.6). Table 1 sets out the average value for calorie intake and the proportional calorie intake of every daily intake from all of the surveyed members of the sample; it shows no statistical differences between sexes. The highest caloric contribution is from lunch (34.5%), followed by dinner (23.5%), breakfast (16%), the mid-afternoon snack (14.5%), and, finally, the mid-morning snack (11.9%).

Figure 1 displays the percentage contribution from the different food groups in relation to daily calorie intake. Cereals (34%), dairy products (19%), and meats (17%) were responsible for approximately 70% of the total caloric intake. Table 2 contains the percentage contributions of the macronutrients and fatty acids to the total calorie intake for every respondent, in order to form a comparison with a healthy diet prototype. Excessive protein intake, mainly from animal origins is observed, as well as a deficient intake of carbohydrates and a higher than recommended intake of fatty acids. The daily average consumption of cholesterol was 315.6±05.9 mg, while total fiber was 26.5±13.5g.

Table 3 shows the average values of the intake of minerals and vitamins. The average value of calcium, iodine, and vitamins A, D, and E were lower than the recommended intakes for minerals and vitamins, respectively.

Table 1. Calorie intake (kilocalories) and calorie percentage contribution (%) of daily meals in the surveyed students

Meal	Calorie intake (Kcal) M (CI 95%)	Calorie contribution (%) M (CI 95%)
Breakfast	323.5 (313.9-333.1)	16.0 (15.5-16.5)
Mid-morning snack	253.8 (242.2-265.4	11.9 (11.4-12.4)
Lunch	734.2 (714.6-753.8)	34.5 (33.7-35.4)
Afternoon snack	298.1 (287.7-308.5)	14.5 (14.0-15.0)
Dinner	498.2 (480.3-516.1)	23.5 (22.8-24.2)

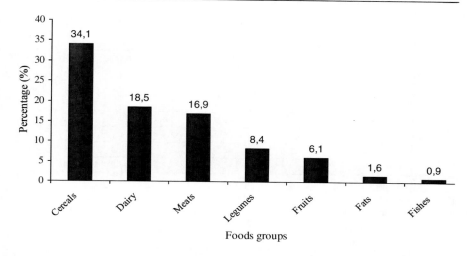

Figure 1. Percentage contribution of the different food groups in relation to daily calorie intake.

Table 2. Percentage contribution of immediate principles and fatty acids to daily calorie intake in the whole group

Nutrients (recommended percentage)	Percentage (%)
Proteins (10-15%)	20.3
Animal origin	64.5
Carbohydrates (50-55%)	48.8
Total fat (30-35%)	30.9
SFA (7-10%)	12.6
MUFA (15-20%)	10.9
PUFA (6-10%)	3.74

Table 3. Daily intake of minerals and vitamins

Nutrients	Total group M (SD)	DRIs
Calcium (mg)	911.7 (174.1)	1300
Iron (mg)	18.3 (6.0)	8
Iodine (µg)	79.2 (22.6)	120
Magnesium (mg)	311.8 (83.3)	240
Zinc (mg)	10.5 (2.7)	8
Selenium (µg)	125.8 (39.6)	40

Table 3. (Continued)

Nutrients	Total group M (SD)	DRIs
Phosphorus (mg)	1606.8 (294.0)	1250
Thiamine (mg)	1.7 (0.5)	0.9
Riboflavin (mg)	1.9 (0.5)	0.9
Niacin (mg)	39.0 (7.6)	12
Vitamin B_6(mg)	2.0 (0.6)	1.0
Folate (µg)	334.6 (150.2)	300
Vitamin B_{12}(mg)	5.8 (2.5)	1.8
Vitamin C (mg)	54.3 (34.3)	45
Vitamin A (µg)	463.6 (204.6)	600
Vitamin D (µg)	88.0 (66.3)	200
Vitamin E (mg)	3.8 (1.7)	11

Percentage Contribution of Food Groups

Table 4 shows the percentage contribution of the different food groups in the daily macronutrient intake. The ingestion of proteins came mainly from meats (38%), cereals (20%), and dairy products (19.7%). Carbohydrates were obtained from cereals (55%); lipids were acquired from dairy products (36.9%) and meats (27.7%). SFA came mainly from dairy products (47.5%), meats (22.4%), and sweets, bakery products, and pastries (18.9%); cholesterol came from meats (42.9%), eggs (21.4%), and dairy products (20.2%). Finally, fiber was consumed from legumes (37.8%), cereals (36.5%), and fruits (16.9%).

Table 5 shows the percentage contribution of the different food groups in relation to the daily mineral intake. The calcium intake came mainly from dairy products (71.8%); iron was accessed in cereals (30.2%), meats (25.1%), and legumes (23.1%); iodine came from dairy products (43.7%), while magnesium was acquired from cereals (26.8%), legumes (25.5%), and dairy products (20.9%). Zinc came from meats (43.5%) and selenium was consumed through cereals (62.4%). Finally, phosphorus primarily came from dairy products (35%) and meats (25.5%).

Table 4. Percentage contribution (%) of the different food groups to daily macronutrient intake

Food group	Dairy	Cereals	Meats	Eggs	Vegetab	Legumes	Fruits	Fishes	Sweets	Fat
Proteins	19.7	20.8	38.0	2.0	0.5	11.5	0.7	2.9	3.9	-
CH	9.0	55.0	2.4	-	0.7	9.1	10.6	-	13.2	-
Fat	36.9	6.4	27.7	3.6	1.9	-	1.4	0.8	15.1	6.2
SFA	47.5	3.2	22.4	2.2	-	-	-	-	18.9	4.3
MUFA	32.4	3.3	33.5	4.8	-	-	1.8	-	14.5	7.8
PUFA	23.8	12.3	27.5	3.9	7.1	-	3.0	1.5	9.9	11.0
Cholest	20.2	-	42.9	21.4	-	-	-	5.4	8.5	1.6
Fiber	-	36.5	-	-	2.4	37.8	16.9	-	6.4	-

Vegetab: Vegetables. CH: Carbohydrates. Cholest.: Cholesterol.

Table 5. Percentage contribution (%) of food groups to daily mineral intake

Food group	Dairy	Cereals	Meats	Eggs	Vegetab	Legumes	Fruits	Fishes	Sweets	Fat
Ca	71.8	11.6	2.4	1.0	4.9	-	1.4	-	5.9	-
Fe	2.7	30.2	25.1	1.9	1.5	23.1	6.6	1.5	7.2	-
I	43.7	16.6	15.5	2.6	2.2	-	2.6	8.6	6.8	1.4
Mg	20.9	26.8	14.0	-	1.6	25.5	4.7	2.4	3.3	-
Zn	19.8	15.0	43.5	2.76	14.2	-	2.1	-	1.8	-
Se	5.1	62.4	14.2	1.2	4.3	-	2.1	7.1	3.6	-
P	35.0	15.2	25.5	2.2	14.0	-	1.6	2.2	4.4	-

Table 6. Percentage contribution (%) of food groups to daily vitamin intake

Food group	Dairy	Cereals	Meats	Eggs	Vegetab	Legumes	Fruits	Fishes	Sweets	Fat
B1	11.2	27.0	29.6	1.3	1.3	17.1	5.3	1.3	6.6	-
B2	41.3	19.4	19.9	3.5	7.0	-	3.5	1.0	5.0	-
Niacin	10.3	25.6	42.5	1.4	9.8	-	0.7	5.7	3.9	-
B6	9.9	21.3	38.0	1.0	1.9	17.6	5.9	1.9	2.8	-
Folate	9.4	30.4	5.3	3.4	4.3	34.9	4.8	1.2	6.3	-
B12	38.3	4.1	38.3	9.4	-	-	-	77	2.3	-
C	9.4	18.4	4.7	-	13.5	-	54.0	-	-	-
A	47.6	11.9	-	9.7	14.1	-	2.4	-	7.2	7.0
D	11.0	43.1	-	17.2	-	-	-	-	8.8	19.9
E	11.4	3.2	6.5	8.4	4.3	24.6	20.8	2.5	6.5	11.2

Table 6 details the percentage contribution from the different food groups to daily vitamin intake. Thiamine (vitamin B1) intake came mainly from meats (29.6%), cereals (27%), and legumes (17%); riboflavin (vitamin B2) came from dairy products (41.3%), meats (19.5%), and cereals (19.4%); niacin was accessed from meats (42.5%), and cereals (25.6%); vitamin B6 came from meats (38%), cereals (21.3%), and legumes (17.6%); folate was consumed in legumes (34.9%) and cereals (30.4%), while vitamin B12 mainly came from dairy products (38.3%) and meats (38.3%). Vitamin A was acquired from dairy products (47.6%) and vitamin C primarily came from fruits (54%) and cereals (18.4%); vitamin D came from cereals (43.1%) and, finally, vitamin E was sourced from legumes (29.8%) and fruits (20.8%).

DISCUSSION

Nutritional surveys based on recall are an optimal and widely used method in cross-sectional studies for descriptive purposes, as in this case [23]. A compendium of food pictures showing servings and sizes was used in order to help the respondents specify the quantity and/or size of the corresponding servings that they had consumed over the previous three days. These pictures allowed both the surveyed students to identify the serving/size and the interviewer to estimate the consumed amounts [20]. These kinds of surveys have important methodological limitations that we have tried to correct. On one hand, the option to include a 24-hour recall would have not adequately considered the intra individual variability of the larger sample; on the other hand, these surveys are somehow dependent on memory and, in addition, especially in this case, on the children's ability to describe the consumed food. That is the reason why the surveyed children were students from 3rd to 6th grade in primary education (9-12 years old).

At present, the clinical validity of BMI as an anthropometric parameter to define nutritional status in childhood and adolescence is admitted [24-26]. Owing to the variability of body composition throughout the pediatric age, specific reference charts are used for different ages and sexes. This nutritional study has used the charts and tables from Ferrandez et al. (Centro Andrea Prader, Zaragoza 2004) as a reference, which are widely used and have proven their utility in this academic environment.

Eating habits of surveyed scholars, all of them having a normal nutritional status, reflected a dietary model that, despite covering caloric needs for the corresponding age, differed slightly from the Mediterranean prototype. On the whole, schoolchildren consumed meats and derivatives almost every day on a recurring basis. Meanwhile, the consumption of vegetables, legumes, and fruits, was considerably lower, while fish consumption was marginal. Dairy products and cereals consumption was relatively limited; however, sweets, bakery products, and pastry consumption was slightly high, being responsible for 13.2% of all carbohydrates consumed. The distribution of caloric intake along the five daily meals was adjusted to the recommended proportional distribution.

An immediate consequence of developing this dietary pattern by schoolchildren in our environment is the evidence of a clear imbalance in the percentage contribution of macronutrients towards the daily caloric intake. Fat intake, even though it is quantitatively sufficient, as it represented 30.9% of total calorie intake, showed an excess in SFA, to the detriment of MUFA and PUFA; in addition, cholesterol dietary intake, especially in males, exceeded the recommended 300 mg per day. Carbohydrate intake barely represented 48.8% of total calorie intake; this means that it did not get to the percentage contribution it should as a main energetic component of the diet at that age. However, protein intake slightly overpassed the established recommendations; it represented 20.3% of total calorie intake. Furthermore, there was a clear imbalance between animal origin and vegetable origin for food; animal protein intake was responsible for two-thirds of total protein intake. Another consequence of this dietary model is the deficient coverage of some minerals and vitamins; in fact, calcium, iodine, vitamin A, D, and E intakes were below the established recommendations in both sexes. This means that the characteristics of this dietary model do not match the basic concept of a balanced diet, since, despite representing an adequate energy intake, it does not guarantee sufficient nutrients in adequate quantities or proportions to achieve an optimal nutritional status.

Another characteristic of a balanced diet is the variety and diversity of foods of which it is made. However, the dietary model of the surveyed students lacked this distinctive feature; in fact, the majority of nutrients were provided, with few exceptions, by the triad: dairy products, cereals, and meats. When analyzing the percentage contribution of the different food groups in nutrient intake, we observe how the intake of proteins, SFA, and cholesterol depended primarily on meats and/or cured meat. Although meat is an essential element in any balanced diet as a source of high-value biological proteins, minerals (iron, zinc and phosphorus), and B-complex vitamins (thiamine, riboflavin, niacin, pyridoxine and cyanocobalamin), it is also a source of SFA (palmitic, stearic, myristic) and cholesterol. That is the reason why it is advisable to limit lean meats and/or poultry consumption to 3-4 servings per week, while fatty meats and/or cured meats should only be consumed occasionally. Likewise, dairy products also contribute substantially to protein, saturated fat, and cholesterol intake, while also representing the main source of calcium, iodine, and vitamin A. However, even though dairy products have a high content of SFA and cholesterol, their consumption should be increased as yogurts and cheeses, with the aim of making up for the deficiency in calcium and, to a lesser extent, vitamin A and iodine in school kids. When a normal nutritional status is reached – as it happened in this case – low fat and/or modified fat composition dairy products should be consumed. Finally, it is remarkable how cereals specifically contribute to calorie intake due to their high complex carbohydrates content. Additionally, they are an important source of protein, which needs to be complemented with other proteins of vegetable and/or animal origin, since they are low biological value proteins, as well as dietary fiber, minerals (iron, magnesium, and selenium), and B-complex vitamins (thiamine, riboflavin, niacin, pyridoxine, and folate). Therefore, while meat consumption should be moderated, cereal intake (breakfast, bread, rice, and pasta) should be encouraged in order to increase, on one hand, its caloric percentage contribution and, on the other hand, to average the origin of protein content in the diet. Furthermore, it would help increase calcium intake and compensate for the hypothetically lower contribution of B-complex vitamins from meats.

Consumption of the rest of the food groups among surveyed students, except for sweets, bakery products, and pastry, was obviously lower and would largely explain the deficient intake in iodine and fat-soluble vitamins (A, D, and E). For example, although the nutritional value of vegetables as a source of macronutrients is limited, with the exception of tubers, which are rich in starch, they are rich in dietary fiber and vitamins A, E, and C. In this way, their daily intake would help correct the deficiency in vitamins inherent in the dietary model for schoolchildren. Legumes should be given an appropriate consideration due to their high content of proteins, dietary fiber, iron, calcium, and vitamin E, as well as their ability to compensate for the hypothetically lower intake of iron and B-complex vitamins that would normally be obtained from meat. Fruits are a low-calorie food group, but they stand out because of their high content of dietary fiber and vitamins A, C, and E. That is why the daily or recurrent intake of fruits would contribute to a high intake in the currently deficient vitamins A and E, in addition to providing phytonutrients with antioxidant properties.

With regards to foods of animal origin and the low-frequency consumption of fish, it should be noted that, generally, they have a low calorie content but contain high-value biological proteins – even higher than those from meat – and PUFA, while also providing water-soluble vitamins (thiamine, riboflavin, and niacin) and fat-soluble vitamins (vitamins A and D). In addition, sea fish and shellfish are the main natural sources of iodine in our diet, as well as valuable sources of calcium, phosphorous, and iron. Therefore, its consumption should be promoted as an essential food in schoolchildren's eating habits. By doing so, a higher intake of iodine, together with iodized salt, PUFA, and vitamins A and D, would be guaranteed and, consequently, it would help improve the deficient intake of these nutrients in schoolchildren.

The consumption of eggs among surveyed schoolchildren corresponds to the recommended frequency (no more than one per day and three per week). The fat content in the yolk is mainly SFA, MUFA, and cholesterol, while the yolk is rich in minerals (iron, calcium, zinc, and selenium), water-soluble vitamins (thiamine, riboflavin, and vitamin B12), and fat-soluble vitamins (vitamins A and D). However, despite this moderated intake, they still noticeably contribute to the cholesterol content of schoolchildren's diet.

Bakery product and pastry intake was very obvious, especially in the breakfast or the afternoon snack of schoolchildren. The nutritional value of pastry products is quite heterogeneous, due to the great variety of ingredients and proportions used. In general, their energy value is very high owing to their composition of refined sugars and fat. For instance, the quantity of SFA depends on the type of vegetable oil used (palm oil or olive oil), while the amount of cholesterol depends on the origin of the fat (lard and butter) or the addition of other ingredients (e.g. eggs). What is recommended is their occasional ingestion and, therefore, it is advisable to substitute sweets, bakery products, and pastries with cereals and fruits, thereby increasing the intake of fiber, minerals, and vitamins, as well as nutrients with functional properties, while noticeably reducing the intake of cholesterol and SFA.

This dietary pattern, together with the data provided by different authors, highlights a tendency in Spanish society to take up new Occidental dietary models, which are characterized by the high intake of proteins and animal fat at the expense of complex carbohydrates [27-36].

We should mention the fact that a normal nutritional status among the schoolchildren in our environment does not guarantee that their dietary model is healthy, as we do find a nutritional imbalance. However, the most relevant finding is that these nutritional deficiencies could be corrected by increasing the consumption of dairy products (milk, yogurt, etc.), cereals (bread, rice, pasta, etc.), legumes, fruits, vegetables, and fish (tuna, sardine, salmon, etc.) intake, coupled with reducing the intake of meat and promoting the use of olive oil as the exclusive culinary oil. In this way, we could guarantee the sufficient intake of all vitamins and minerals that are deficient in the dietary model of the surveyed schoolchildren.

An important conclusion emerged from this chapter: it is imperative to design nutritional education programs with the goal of helping the general population, schoolchildren in particular, become aware and ready to begin healthy eating. In order to do this, public authorities should coordinate enough human and/or material resources to keep following our traditional eating habits and make them compatible with the new lifestyles of modern societies, encouraging nutritional counseling in primary healthcare, and developing nutritional education programs in educational institutions. In this way, schoolchildren would have an excellent means to prevent disease and promote health after completing their compulsory education.

REFERENCES

[1]   Serra-Majem L, Roman B, Estruch R. Scientific evidence of interventions using the Mediterranean diet: a systematic review. *Nutr Rev* 2006; 64: S27-S47.

[2]   Helsing E. Traditional diets and disease patterns of the mediterranean, circa 1960. *Am J Clin Nutr* 1995; 61 (Suppl): 1329-1337.

[3]   Willet WC, Sacks F, Trichopoulou A, Drescher G, Ferro-Luzzi A, Helsing E, Trichopoulou D. Mediterranean diet pyramid: a cultural model for healthy eating. *Am J Clin Nutr* 1995; 61 (Suppl): 1402-1406.

[4]   Trichopoulou A, Lagiou P. Healthy traditional mediterranean diet: an expression of culture, history, and lifestyle. *Nutr Rev* 1997; 55: 383-389.

[5]   Sánchez-Villegas A, Bes-Rastrollo M, Martinez-Gonzalez MA, Serra-Majem L. Adherence to a mediterranean dietary pattern and weight gain in a follow-up study: the SUN cohort. *Int J Obes* 2006; 30: 350-358.

[6]   Trichopoulou A, Costacou T, Bamia C, Trichopoulos D. Adherence to a mediterranean diet and survival in a greek population. *New Engl J Med* 2003; 348: 2599-2608.

[7]   Tur JA, Serra-Majem L, Romaguera D, Pons A. Does the diet of the Balearic population, a mediterranean type diet, still provide adequate antioxidant nutrient intakes? *Eur J Nutr* 2005; 44: 204-213.

[8]   Moreno LA, Sarria A, Popkin BM. The nutrition transition in Spain: a european Mediterranean country. *Eur J Clin Nutr* 2002; 56: 992-1003.

[9]   Tur JA, Romaguera D, Pons A. Food consumption patterns in a mediterranean region: does the mediterranean diet still exist? *Ann Nutr Metab* 2004; 48: 193-201.

[10] Bach-Faig A, Berry EM, Lairon D, Reguant J, Trichopoulou A, Dernini S, Medina FX, Battino M, Belahsen R, Miranda G, Serra-Majem L. Mediterranean diet pyramid today. Science and cultural updates. *Public Health Nutr* 2011; 14: 2274-2284.

[11] Ferrara LA, Raimondi S, d´Episcopo L, Guida L, Dello Russo A, Marotta T. Olive oil and reduced need for antihypertensive medications. *Arch Intern Med* 2000; 160: 837-842.

[12] Kris-Etherton P, Eckel RH, Howard BV, Jeor S, Bazzarre TL. AHA Science Advisory: Lyon diet heart study. Benefits of a mediterranean-style, national cholesterol education program/american heart association step I dietary pattern on cardiovascular disease. *Circulation* 2001; 103: 1823-1825.

[13] Hu FB. The Mediterranean diet and mortality–olive oil and beyond. *New Engl J Med* 2003; 348: 2595-2596.

[14] Trichopoulou A, Naska A, Antoniou A, Friel S, Trygg K, Turrini A. Vegetable and fruit: the evidence in their favour and the public health perspective. *Int J Vitam Nutr Res* 2003; 73: 63-69.

[15] Estruch R, Martinez-González MA, Corella D, Salas-Salvadó J, Ruiz-Gutiérrez V, Covas MI, Fiol M, Gómez-Gracia E, López-Sabater MC, Vinyoles E. et al. Effects of a mediterranean-style diet on cardiovascular risk factors: a randomized trial. *Ann Intern Med* 2006; 145: 1-11.

[16] Gil A, Ortega RM, Maldonado J. Wholegrain cereals and bread: a duet of the Mediterranean diet for the prevention of chronic diseases. *Public Health Nutr* 2011; 14: 2316-2322.

[17] Van den Brandt PA. The impact of a Mediterranean diet and healthy lifestyle on premature mortality in men and women. *Am J Clin Nutr* 2011; 94: 913-920.

[18] Kontou N, Psaltopoulou T, Panagiotakos D, Dimopoulos MA, Linos A. The mediterranean diet in cancer prevention: a review. *J Med Food* 2011; 14: 1065-1078.

[19] Kastorini CM, Milionis HJ, Esposito K, Giugliano D, Goudevenos J.A.; Panagiotakos DB. The effect of Mediterranean diet on metabolic syndrome and its components: a meta-analysis of 50 studies and 534,906 individuals. *J Am Coll Cardiol* 2011: 57: 1299-1313.

[20] SUVIMAX. Portions Alimentaires. Manuel photos pourl'estimation des quantités. Paris: *Polytechnica*. 2002.

[21] Programa de cálculo nutricional CESNID 1.0 (CD-ROM). Centre d'Ensenyament Superior de Nutrició i Dietética. Universitat de Barcelona-*McGraw-Hill:* Barcelona, 2003.

[22] Dietary References Intakes: Macronutrients, Elements and vitamins. Food and Nutrition Board, Institute of Medicine, National Academy of Sciences, 2004. http://www.nap.edu25

[23] Martínez MA, Alonso A, Egües N. Sistemas de evaluación del consumo de alimentos. In: Nutrición aplicada y dietoterapia; Muñoz M., Aranceta J., García-Jalón I., Eds. EUNSA: Pamplona, 2004, pp. 67-82

[24] Reilly JJ, Dorosty AR, Emmett PM. Identification of the obese child: adequacy of the body mass index for clinical practice and epidemiology. *Int J Obes* 2000; 24: 1623–1627.

[25] Marrodán-Serrano MD, Mesa-Santurino MS, Alba-Díaz JA, Ambrosio-Soblechero B, Barrio-Caballero PA, Drak-Hernández L, Gallardo-Yepes M, Lermo-Castelar J, Rosa-Rosa JM, González-Montero de Espinosa M. Obesity screening: updated criteria and their clinical and populational validity. *An Pediatr* (Barc) 2006; 65: 5–14.

[26] Calañas-Continente A, Arrizabalaga J, Caixàs A, Cordido F. Diagnostic and therapeutic recommendations for overweight and obesity during adolescence. *Med Clin* (Barc) 2010; 135: 265–273.

[27] Rodriguez-Artalejo F, Banegas JR, Graciani MA, Hernández-Vecino R, Rey-Calero J. Food and nutrient consumption in Spain in the period 1940-1988. Analysis of its consistency with the Mediterranean diet. *Med Clin* (Barc) 1996; 106: 161-168.

[28] Iturbe A, Emparanza J, Perales A. Dietary pattern of adolescents in Guipuzcoa. *An Esp Pediatr* 1999; 50: 471-478.

[29] Serra-Majem L, García-Closas R, Ribas L, Pérez-Rodrigo C, Aranceta J. Food patterns of spanish schoolchildren and adolescents: The enKid study. *Public Health Nutrition* 2001; 4: 1433-1438.

[30] Durá-Travé T. Energy and nutrient intake in compulsory high school students. An Esp Pediatr 2001, 54, 547-554.

[31] Aranceta J. Spanish food patterns. *Public Health Nutr* 2001; 4: 1399-1402.

[32] Sánchez-Villegas A, Martinez JA, De Irala J, Martínez-González MA. Determinants of the adherence to an a priori defined Mediterranean dietary pattern. *Eur J Nutr* 2002; 41: 249-257.

[33] Serra-Majem L, Ribas L, Ngo J, Ortega R.M, García A, Pérez-Rodrigo C, Aranceta J. Food, Youth and the Mediterranean diet in Spain. Development of KIDMED, Mediterranean Diet Quality Index in children and adolescents. *Public Health Nutrition* 2004; 7: 931-935.

[34] Mariscal-Arcas M, Rivas A, Velasco J, Ortega M, Caballero AM, Olea-Serrano F. Evaluation of the Mediterranean Diet Quality Index (KIDMED) in children and adolescents in Southern Spain. *Public Health Nutrition* 2009; 12: 1408–1412.

[35] Velasco J, Mariscal-Arcas M, Rivas A, Caballero ML, Hernández-Elizondo J, Olea-Serrano F. Assessment of the diet of school children from Granada and influence of social factors. *Nutr Hosp* 2009; 24: 193-199.

[36] Ayechu A, Durá T. Quality of dietary habits (adherence to a mediterranean diet) in pupils of compulsory secondary education. *An Sist Sanit Navar* 2010; 33: 35-42.

In: Focus on Nutrition …
Editor: Teodoro Durá-Travé

ISBN: 978-1-63463-223-2
© 2015 Nova Science Publishers, Inc.

Chapter 6

TRACKING OF OVERWEIGHT AND OBESITY IN CHILDHOOD AND ITS IMPACT ON ADOLESCENTS

Teodoro Durá-Travé[1,2], Fidel Gallinas-Victoriano[2],
Monserrat Elso-Fabregas[2], Mikel Mendizábal-Diez[2],
Izaskun Naberan-Mardaras[2]
and Ana Navedo de las Heras[1]
[1]Department of Pediatrics, Faculty of Medicine,
University of Navarra, Pamplona, Spain
[2]Department of Pediatrics, Navarra Hospital Complex,
Pamplona, Spain

ABSTRACT

Objective: To estimate the prevalence of excess body fat in a cohort of children aged 2 to 14 years, and calculate the risk of overweight during adolescence when it was present in previous years.

Subjects and method: This was a retrospective study and review of clinical records including weight, height and body mass index in a cohort of 840 children at ages 2, 3, 4, 6, 8, 10, 12 and 14 years. The excess of body fat was calculated following the International Obesity Task Force criteria and showing the odds ratio of having overweight at age 14 years when it was present in any previous year.

Results: The prevalence of overweight at age 2 was 8.5%, increased progressively to 32.6% at age 8, and then decreased to 22.5% at age 14. The prevalence of overweight was significantly higher (p < 0.05) in females at age 2 and 3 years and lower (p < 0.05) at age 12 and 14 with respect to males. The probability of presenting overweight/obesity in adolescence was 15 times higher when overweight was present at age 8.

Conclusions: This chapter shows that overweight at any pediatric age implies a high risk of overweight/obesity in adolescence.

INTRODUCTION

The prevalence of excess body weight (overweight and obesity) in children has progressively increased in industrialized countries, to the point that it represents the most relevant nutritional disorder in our environment [1-3] at present day. In addition, excess body weight will remain in adulthood for most teenagers; this fact justifies, on one side, the interests to know the magnitude of the problem in order to take effective preventive and/or therapeutic measures and, on the other side, the need to be considered as a major public health issue given the labor, social, economic and sanitary consequences [4-7].

However, despite its epidemic characteristics and health significance, there are no uniform methodological criteria that allow an accurate diagnosis of excess body weight; the published epidemiological data are, consequently, quite variable, and this complicates the fulfillment of international –or even national - comparisons [8-10]. At present day, the clinical validity of body mass index (BMI) as an anthropometric variable to define overweight and obesity is admitted [11-14]; in the same way, the charts proposed by Cole et al. [15], which have been supported by the *International Obesity Task Force (IOTF)*, have been recommended as international reference standards and gather anthropometric data from different ethnic groups.

Most of the published studies on the prevalence of child overweight and obesity, both in national as well as international scope, are cross-sectional studies [8-9]; there are few cohort studies that allow, for instance, estimating the predictive value that excess body weight in early stages of life may have on the nutritional status in later stages and, therefore, setting the most appropriate time to start a preventive and/or curative intervention presumably prior to a consolidation of a state of overweight or obesity [16-17].

The aim of this chapter is to estimate the prevalence of excess body weight in a cohort of children who are evaluated from 2 to 14 years of age, by applying the international standards of the IOFT, as well as to calculate the risk of excess body weight at age 14 in those patients who showed this nutritional status at earlier stages.

MATERIAL AND METHODS

The institutionalized Program for Child Care in the Community of Navarre includes periodic health examinations during the first year of life and at ages 1, 2, 3, 4, 6, 8, 10, 12 and 14 years. The clinical and anthropometric (weight and height) data are consistently registered in chronological order in the clinical records of each patient.

This infrastructure of the Health Service enabled us to obtain a sample of patients by applying stratified sampling proportional to the distribution of child population in the three Health Areas existing in Navarra: Pamplona (75.7%), Tudela (14.6%) and Estella (9.7%) (National Institute of Statistics, Spain). To obtain sub-samples corresponding to each Health Area, considering that every Primary Care pediatrician attends similar child population, we required the cooperation of a random selection of 25 pediatricians (18 from the Health Area of Pamplona, 4 from the Health Area of Tudela and 3 from the Health Area of Estella). These health professionals should review a random selection of clinical records of 50 patients (25 males and 25 females) who were born in 1993 and collect the registered weight and heights of every periodic health examination.

This sequence contributed with anthropometric data from 876 patients provided by 21 pediatricians, and 36 cases (4.1%) were not accepted because of a significant lack of data (less than six periodic examinations correctly fulfilled). Therefore, the total number of patients who were included in this study was 840 (437 males and 403 females). Of the total sample, 630 patients (75%) coming from the Health Area of Pamplona, 131 (15.6%) from the Health Area of Tudela and 79 (9.4%) from the Health Area of Estella.

All measurements were performed by trained observers (pediatric nurse practitioners) from the Pediatric office of the previously cited Health Centers. Every patient was placed in underwear and barefoot. An Añó-Sayol® scale with a reading range of 0 to 120 kg and a precision of 100 g was used for measuring weight and a height rigid rod ranging 60 to 120 cm and with 0.1 cm precision for measuring height.

BMI was calculated according to the following formula: weight (kg) / height2 (m). The international charts from Cole et al.(IOTF)[18] were used for the evaluation of the prevalence of excess body weight (overweight and obesity); they set BMI cut off points for overweight and obesity among 2 and 18 years of age by extrapolating the adult values that have been proposed by the WHO (25 and 30 kg/m2, respectively). Therefore, only anthropometric data corresponding to 2 to 14 years were considered. The odds ratio (OR) – stratifying by sex – of suffering from excess body weight (overweight/obesity) at age 14 among those patients who showed this condition in preceding ages was calculated. In order to facilitate its comprehension, the OR has been changed into likelihood using the formula: OR/OR+1.

Results are displayed as means and percentages with the corresponding confidence intervals (95% CI). Statistical analysis (comparison of proportions and binary logistic regression) was carried out using the *Statistical Packages for the Social Sciences* (SPSS) software, version 17.0 for Windows (Chicago, Illinois, USA). Statistical significance was assumed when the p value was less than 0.05.

RESULTS

Periodic Health examinations in Navarre corresponding to the Child and Adolescents Care Program usually are usually set to coincide with the birth date of the patients. Table 1 shows the distribution of the sample by age and sex.

Table 1. Distribution of the sample according to age and sex

Age Years (CI 95%)	Males	Females	Total
2.01 (1.97-2.05)	412	374	786
3.03 (2.96-3.09)	373	338	711
4.04 (3.97-4.12)	367	358	725
6.05 (6.04-6.06)	388	382	770
8.03 (8.02-8.04)	350	332	682
10.06 (10.5-10.7)	367	369	736
12.08 (12.07-12.09)	274	257	531
14.08 (14.06-14.09)	307	297	604

Figure 1 displays the prevalence of excess body weight of the entire sample in every age considered. The prevalence of excess body weight at age 2 is 8.5%, increases progressively up to the maximum level (32.6%) at age 8 and then decreases later down to 22.5% at age 14.

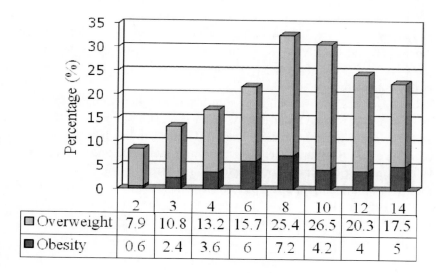

	2	3	4	6	8	10	12	14
▢Overweight	7.9	10.8	13.2	15.7	25.4	26.5	20.3	17.5
■Obesity	0.6	2.4	3.6	6	7.2	4.2	4	5

Age (years)

Figure 1. Prevalence of excess body weight (overweight and obesity).

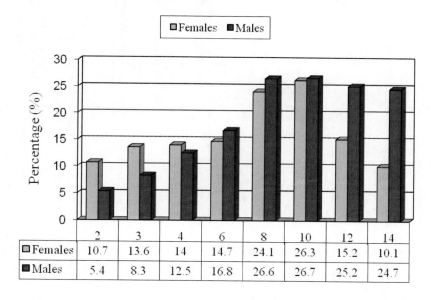

	2	3	4	6	8	10	12	14
▢Females	10.7	13.6	14	14.7	24.1	26.3	15.2	10.1
■Males	5.4	8.3	12.5	16.8	26.6	26.7	25.2	24.7

Figure 2. Prevalence of overweight in both sexes.

The highest prevalence rate of overweight arises at age 10 (26.5%) and obesity at age 8 (7.2%). Subsequently, these rates decrease and the prevalence of overweight and obesity is 17.5% and 5% at age 14, respectively. Figure 2 presents and compares the prevalence rates of overweight for both sexes in every age considered.

The prevalence of overweight is significantly higher (p<0.05) in females at age 2 and 3 years and significantly lower (p<0.05) at age 12 and 14 with respect to males. There are no significant differences in the distribution among sexes at ages 4, 6, 8 and 10 years. Figure 3 sets out and compares the prevalence rates of obesity for both sexes in the different ages. The prevalence of obesity is significantly higher (p<0.05) in females at age 4 and significantly lower (p<0.05) at 10, 12 and 14 years of age with respect to males. No significant differences were observed at ages 2, 3, 6 and 8 years.

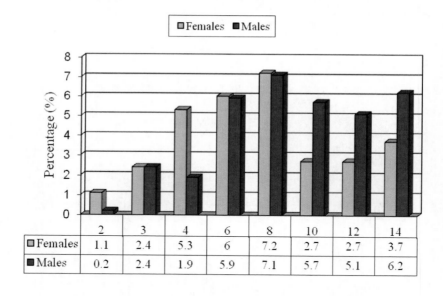

Figure 3. Prevalence of obesity in both sexes.

Table 2 illustrates the odds ratio for the nutrition situation of excess body weight (overweight/obesity) at age 14 for both sexes whenever it was present in any previous age.

There is an increase in the value of the odds ratio with age and, therefore, an increased likelihood to present excess body weight at age 14 whenever this nutritional status was present in previous ages. Even when an excess body weigh in preschool children (2, 3 and 4 years old) already implies a significant risk (p<0.05) of retaining this nutrition status at age 14, the presence of excess body weight at age 8 (the period of maximum prevalence) is related to a probability 15 times higher of maintaining this status at age 14, in both sexes, compared to the absence of excess weight.

Table 2. Odds ratio for the presence of excess body weight at age 14 in relation to the same condition in early ages

Age (years)	Males* OR (IC 95%)	Females* OR (IC 95%)
2	6.61 (2.4-18.3)	5.23 (2.6-10.5)
3	7.83 (3.6-17.1)	4.16 (1.6-6.1)
4	8.75 (4.2-18.1)	9.48 (4.9-18.1)
6	9.21 (4.5-18.8)	4.64 (1.04-0.7)
8	15.49 (7.2-33.3)	15.88 (3.7-67.3)
10	14.17 (6.9-28.9)	16.61 (6.4-42.9)

(*) Every *p* value was lower than 0.05.

Therefore, as for males, the probability of presenting with excess weight at age 14 after showing this status at ages 2, 3, 4 and 6 years is 86.8%, 88.6%, 89.7% and 90.2%, respectively; and the probability after showing excess weight at ages 8 and 10 is 93.9% and 93.6%, respectively. As for females, the probability of suffering from excess weight at age 14 after presenting this condition at ages 2, 3, 4 and 6 is 83.9%, 80.6%, 89.7% and 90.4%, respectively; and the probability after presenting this status at ages 8 and 10 is 94.1% and 94.3%, respectively.

DISCUSSION

The choice of reference standards constitutes a determining factor in the evaluation of nutritional status. British [19] and French [20] charts have been used in our country until the publication of growth charts from Hernández et al.[21] which have had a wide diffusion and proved clinical usefulness. The need to update the reference charts in pursuance of being adapted to the secular growth trend explains the succession of anthropometric studies that have been performed in different national and foreign populations or communities [22-25]. At present day, the most updated charts for classification of pediatric population by weight are those from Serra-Majem et al.(Enkid study) [26 and the *Estudio español de crecimiento 2008* from Carrascosa el al. [27]. With regard to these national references, we should note how both, as the authors themselves remark, reveal a disproportionate increase in the values corresponding to upper percentiles, which define overweight and obesity, regarding qualified international references [15, 28, 29]. This fact is probably due to the inclusion of patients with excess body weight in the process, which has been explicitly avoided when developing the international standards. Therefore, national references tend to undervalue the problem of overweight and obesity and, consequently, the clinical applicability is questionable. On the other hand, the most frequently used international references correspond to the charts by the *Center for Disease Control and Prevention* (CDC, 2000) [28], as well as those by Cole et al. (IOTF) [15] and WHO (*WHO Reference 2007*) [29]; however, the need to standardize methodological criteria in the evaluation of nutritional status has led several expert committees to consider the cut off points proposed by Cole as useful to define overweight and obesity. These references, which have been criticized by some authors [11,30], have gradually gained in clinical relevance and support by the scientific community, and this enables, on one side, to make comparisons among the results of the different national and international studies [10, 31-33], and, on the other side, justifies the use as reference standards in this chapter.

The comparison of the prevalence rates of excess body weight in child population in Navarre with the data provided by the different national and international cross-sectional studies that have been published in the last decade (whose methodology is similar after applying the standards from the IOTF (table 3), shows that the prevalence rate of excess weight in our environment is similar to that from other Spanish regions [11, 31, 34], countries of the Mediterranean area [10, 35] and the United States of America [36], and it is higher than the rates from central European countries [15, 30, 33-38]. The validation and application of common methodological references, such as the international standards supported by the IOTF, would help calculate the overall magnitude of this problem and, consequently, program and develop preventive strategies which can be adapted to the assistance requirements of every country or region.

Cohort studies, due to the longitudinal nature, offer a series of advantages. On one hand, they register the temporary sequence of the development of a concrete disturbance and, in this case, the excess body weight. The obtained data show how the prevalence of excess weight gains further significance in preschool age, especially in females, when 16.8% (one out of six patients) of patients present with excess body weight at age 4 years.

Table 3. Prevalence of excess body weight (overweight and obesity) in national and international studies when applying the references from the IOTF

Reference	Origin	Group of age	Prevalence
Caroli et al, 2001[10]	Italy	9 years	36.0
Krassas et al, 2001[35]	Greece	6-10 years	30.9
		11-17 years	21.6
Wang et al, 2002[36]	Brazil	6-9 years	13.9
	China	6-9 years	7.7
	Russia	6-9 years	9.0
	USA	6-9 years	25.6
Rolland-Cachera et al, 2002[37]	Paris (France)	7 years; M/F	19.7/18.6
		8 years; M/F	15.6/19.5
		9 years; M/F	18.4/16.9
Lobstein et al, 2003[38]	London (UK)	7-11 years; M/F	22.8/17.0
Zimmermann et al, 2004[30]	Switzerland	6-8 years; M/F	20.4/23.9
		9-10 years; M/F	23.7/22.9
		11-12 years; M/F	17.0/21.5
Marrodan et al, 2006[11]	Madrid (Spain)	6-12 years; M/F	27.6/31.8
		13-20 years; M/F	23.5/17.4
Johannsson et al, 2006[16]	Ireland	6 years; M/F	16.2/23.0
		9 years; M/F	22.9/22.6
Larrañaga et al, 2007[31]	Basque Country (Spain)	4-6 years	29.4
		7-10 years	32.6
		11-14 years	29.9
F. Martinez et al, 2008[34]	Cuenca (Spain)	9-10 years; M/F	29.7/32.0
Péneau et al, 2009[39]	France	6-10 years	14.0
		11-15 years	16.8

M: male. F: female.

Subsequently, the prevalence rate increases and reaches the highest rate at age 8, when 32.6% (one out of three) show excess body weight. Finally, there is a slight decrease during adolescence, at the expense of females, since males do not vary this rate. This means, excess body weight is a nosological entity that begins in early stages of life when diet depends – almost exclusively – on family dietary habits and feeding preferences; this condition then aggravates at the time of school attendance, probably with the acquisition of a certain degree of personal autonomy in feeding since usually some of the intakes take place out of their own houses, in school canteens, or without family supervision. However, a slight improvement is noted, exclusively in females, probably related to negative social connotations that excess weight has in this period of life and that could condition, to a great extent, an increased motivation in female adolescents to make a special effort in order to reverse the upward trend of weight in pediatric age. On the other hand, cohort studies allow estimating the predictive value that excess body weight in early stages has on nutritional status at older ages, such as adolescence [16, 17, 39, 40]. In other words, it is a way to identify patients at risk of developing overweight/obesity during adolescence and, in this way, to ensure early intervention so as to slow the progression of excess weight that could lead to obesity with associated morbidity in adolescents or adults. Accordingly, the obtained data indicate that those who present excess weight in school age, particularly at 8 years, are 15 times more likely to maintain this situation in adolescence, compared to those who do not show this condition; however, excess weight in preschool age in itself implies a significant risk of keeping in this condition in adolescence. These results suggest that excess body weight at any pediatric age, but especially in school age, represents a high-risk situation for overweight/obesity in adolescence and, consequently, in adulthood. Therefore, it is essential to develop preventive strategies that, on one hand, enable to detect child excess weight as soon as possible through an efficient interpretation of anthropometric variables of the corresponding periodic health examinations, and, on the other hand, provide sufficient resources to develop validated programs that include, together with the corresponding dietary restrictions, education activities that promote healthy feeding habits and lifestyle [41].

As a conclusion, the registration of anthropometric data in the regular health examination constitutes a basic preventive activity in such a prevalent health problem; the detection, at any age, of excess of body fat would be the appropriate moment to consider an educational and/or nutritional intervention in order to reduce the risk of overweight/obesity in adolescence and adulthood.

REFERENCES

[1]   Odgen CL, Flegal KM, Carroll, MD, Jhonson CL. Prevalence and trends in overweight among US children and adolescents, 1999-2000. *JAMA* 2002; 288:1728-32.

[2]   Tzotzas T, Krassas GE. Prevalence and trends of obesity in children and adults of South Europe. *Pediatr Endocrinol Rev* 2004; 1 (3 Suppl):448-54.

[3]   Schober E, Rami B, Kirchengast S, Waldhör T, Sefranek R. Recent trend in overweight and obesity in male adolescents in Austria: a population-based study. *Eur J Pediat* 2007; 166:709-14.

[4]   Freedman DS, Khan LF, Serdula MK, Dietz WH, Srinivasan SR, Berenson GS. The relation of childhood BMI to adult adiposity: The Bogalusa Heart Study. *Pediatrics* 2005; 115: 22-7.

[5]   Biro FM, Wien M. Childhood obesity and adult morbidities. *Am J Clin Nutr* 2010; 91:1499-505.

[6]   Field AE, Cook NR, Gillman MW. Weight status in childhood as a predictor of becoming overweight or hypertensive in early adulthood. *Obes Res* 2005; 13:163-9.

[7]   Viner RM, Cole TJ. Adult socioeconomic, educational, social, and psychological outcomes of childhood obesity: a national birth cohort study. *BMJ* 2005; 330:1354-8.

[8]   Livingstone B. Epidemiology of childhood obesity in Europe. *Eur. J. Pediatr* 2000; 159 (1 Suppl): 14-34.

[9]   Serra L, Ribas L, Aranceta J, Pérez C, Saavedra P, Peña L. Childhood and adolescent obesity in Spain. Results of the enKid study (1998-2000). *Med Clin (*Barc) 2003; 21:725-32.

[10] Lobstein T, Frelut ML. Prevalence of overweight among children in *Europe. Obes Rev* 2003; 4:195-200.

[11] Marrodán MD, Mesa MS, Alba JA, Ambrosio B, Barrio PA, Drack L, et al.Obesity screening: updated criteria and their clinical and populational validity. *An Pediatr* (Barc) 2006; 65:5-14.

[12] Dietz WH, Bellizzi M. Introduction: the use of body mass index to assess obesity in children. *Am J Clin Nutr* 1999; 70(suppl):123S–5S.

[13] Reilly JJ, Dorosty AR, Emmett PM. Identification of the obese child: adequacy of the body mass index for clinical practice and epidemiology. *Int J Obes* 2000; 24:1623-27.

[14] Calañas-Continente A, Arrizabalaga JJ, Caixàs A, Cordido F y Grupo de Trabajo sobre Obesidad (SEEN). Diagnostic and therapeutic recommendations for overweight and obesity during adolescence. *Med Clin* (Barc) 2010; 135:265-273.

[15] Cole TJ, Bellizzi MC, Flegal KM, Dietz WH. Establishing a standard definition for child overweight and obesity worldwide: international survey. *BMJ* 2000; 320:1240-5.

[16] Johannsson E, Arngrimsson SA, Thorsdottir I, Sveinsson T. Tracking of overweight from early childhood to adolescence in cohorts born 1988 and 1994: overweight in a high birth weight population. *Int J Obes* (Lond) 2006; 30:1265-71.

[17] Wright CM, Emmett PM, Ness AR, Reilly JJ, Sherriff A. Tracking of obesity and body fatness through mid-childhood. *Arch Dis Child* 2010; 95:612-7.

[18] Tanner J, Whitehouse R. Clinical longitudinal standards for height, weight, height velocity and weight velocity and stages of puberty. *Arch Dis Child* 1976; 51:170–9.

[19] Sempé M, Pèdron G, Roy-Pernot MP. Auxologie. Mèthode et sèquences. Paris. Théraplix. 1979.

[20] Hernández M, Castellet J, Narvaiza JL, Rincón JM, Ruiz I, Sánchez E, et al. Curvas y Tablas de Crecimiento. Instituto de investigación sobre crecimiento y desarrollo. Fundación F. Orbegozo. Ediciones Garsi. Madrid. 1988.

[21] Durá T, Garralda, I, Hualde J. y Grupo Colaborador de Navarra. Longitudinal study of child growth in Navarre (1993-2007). *An Pediatr* (Barc) 2009; 70:526-33.

[22] Fredriks AM, Van Buuren S, Burgmeijer RJ, Meulmeester JF, Benker RJ, Brugman E. Continuing positive secular growth change in the Netherlands 1955–1997. *Pediatr Res* 2000; 47:316-23.

[23] Albertsson-Wikland K, Luo ZC, Niklasson A, Karlberg J. Swedish population-based longitudinal reference values from birth to 18 years of age for height, weight and head circumference. *Acta Paediatr* 2002; 91:739-54.

[24] Karlberg J, Kwan CW, Albertsson-Wikland K. Reference values for change in body mass index from birth to 18 years of age. *Acta Paediatr* 2003; 92:648-52.

[25] Deheeger M, Rolland-Cachera MF. Étude longitudinale de la croissance d'enfants parisiens suivis de l'âge de10 mois à 18 ans. *Arch Pediatr* 2004; 11:1130–44.

[26] Serra-Majem L, Aranceta J, Pérez C, Moreno B, Tojo R, Delgado A, et al. Curvas de referencia para la tipificación ponderal. Población Infantil y Juvenil. Madrid. IM&C,SA. 2002.

[27] Carrascosa A, Fernández JM, Fernández C, Fernández A, López-Siguero JP, Sánchez E, et al. Spanish cross-sectional growth study 2008. Height, weight and body mass index values from birth to adulthood. *An Pediatr* (Barc) 2008; 68:552–69.

[28] The 2000 CDC Growth Charts. Clinical Growth Charts. Available at URL:http://www.cdc.gov/growthcharts/clinical_charts.htm

[29] The WHO Child Growth Standards Growth reference data for 5-19 years.Available at URL: http://www.who.int/growthref/en/

[30] Zimmermann MB, Gübeli C, Püntener C, Molinari L. Detection of overweight and obesity in a national sample of 6-12-y-old Swiss children: accuracy and validity of reference values for body mass index from the US Centers for Disease Control and Prevention and the International Obesity Task Force. *Am. J Clin Nutr* 2004; 79:838-43.

[31] Larrañaga N, Amiano P, Arrizabalaga JJ, Bidaurrazaga J, Gorostiza E. Prevalence of obesity in 4-18-year-old population in the Basque Country, Spain. *Obes Rev* 2007; 8:281-7.

[32] Martínez F, Salcedo F, Rodríguez F, Martínez V, Domínguez L, Torrijos R. Obesity prevalence and tracking of body mass index after a 6 years follow up study in children and adolescents: the Cuenca Study, Spain. *Med Clin* (Barc) 2002; 119:327-30.

[33] Tokmakidis SP, Kasambalis A, Christodoulos AD. Fitness levels of Greek primary schoolchildren in relationship to overweight and obesity. *Eur J Pediatr* 2006; 165:867-74.

[34] Martínez V, Sánchez M, Moya P, Solera M, Notario B, Salcedo F, et al. Trends in excess weight and thinness among Spanish schoolchildren in the period 1992-2004: the Cuenca study. *Public Health Nutr* 2009; 12:1015-8.

[35] Krassas GE, Tzotzas T, Tsametis C, Konstantinidis T. Prevalence and trends in overweight and obesity among children and adolescents in Thessaloniki, Greece. *J Pediatr Endocrinol Metab* 2001;14 (5 Suppl): 1319-26.

[36] Wang Y, Monteiro C, Popkin BM. Trends of obesity and underweight in older children and adolescents in the United States, Brazil, China, and Russia. *Am J Clin Nutr* 2002; 75:971-7.

[37] Rolland-Cachera MF, Castetbon K, Arnault N, Bellisle F, Romano MC, Lehingue Y, et al. Body mass index in 7-9-y-old French children: frequency of obesity, overweight and thinness. *Int J Obes Relat Metab Disord* 2002; 26:1610-6.

[38] Lobstein TJ, James WP, Cole TJ. Increasing levels of excess weight among children in England. *Int J Obes Relat Metab Disord* 2003; 27:1136-8.

[39] Péneau S, Salanave B, Maillard-Teyssier L, Rolland-Cachera MF, Vergnaud AC, Méjean C, et al. Prevalence of overweight in 6- to 15-year-old children in central/western France from 1996 to 2006: trends toward stabilization. *Int J Obes* (Lond). 2009; 33:401-7.

[40] Nader PR, O'Brien M, Houts R, Bradley R, Belsky J, Crosnoe R, et al. Identifying risk for obesity in early childhood. *Pediatrics* 2006; 118:e594-601.

[41] Gussinyer S, García-Reyna NI, Carrascosa A, Gussinyer M, Yeste D, Clemente M, Albisu M. Anthropometric, dietetic and psychological changes after application of the "Niñ@s en movimiento" program in childhood obesity. *Med Clin* (Barc) 2008; 131:245-9.

In: Focus on Nutrition …
Editor: Teodoro Durá-Travé

ISBN: 978-1-63463-223-2
© 2015 Nova Science Publishers, Inc.

Chapter 7

THE CONTRIBUTION OF MILK AND DAIRY PRODUCTS TO NUTRIENT INTAKE IN CHILDREN (9-12 YEARS) AND ADOLESCENTS (13-16 YEARS)

Teodoro Durá-Travé[1,2], Fidel Gallinas-Victoriano[2],
Isabel San Martín-García[2], Ibone Vaquero-Iñigo[2]
and Aida González-Benavides[2]
[1]Department of Pediatrics, Faculty of Medicine,
University of Navarra, Pamplona, Spain
[2]Department of Pediatrics, Navarra Hospital Complex,
Pamplona, Spain

ABSTRACT

Objective: To make a descriptive study of milk and dairy product intake in a population of schoolchildren and adolescents, in addition to analyzing its nutritional contribution to the diet of this population.

Methods: A nutritional survey was carried out in the form of personal interviews (food intake registration on 3 consecutive school days) in a sample of 353 schoolchildren, aged 9 to 12, and 406 adolescents, aged 13 to 16, in Pamplona, Spain.

Results: Dairy product intake was reported by 94% of the respondents in their breakfast, 69.3% in dinner, 42.1% in lunch, 23.3% in their afternoon snack, and 16.4% in their mid-morning snack (there were no statistically significant differences between the age groups). The mean number of dairy product servings was 2.0, being higher (p<0.05) among adolescents (2.22) as compared to schoolchildren (1.75). Milk and dairy products constitute the main sources of calcium, iodine, magnesium, and phosphorous, as well as riboflavin, vitamin B12, and vitamin A. Milk and dairy products also contribute substantially to the daily intake of calories, proteins, potassium, and zinc; however, they also provide significant amounts of saturated fat and cholesterol.

Conclusions: The intake of milk and derivatives in the child/juvenile population is inappropriate. The need to undertake a massive public enlightenment campaign to increase the awareness of families regarding the nutritional importance of this food group should be considered.

INTRODUCTION

Approximately 90% of the body's calcium is stored in bone tissue and the remaining 10% is distributed among the soft tissue and extracellular fluid. The acquisition of optimal bone mass is basically conditioned by the dietary intake of calcium and physical activity. A positive mineral balance for calcium during childhood and adolescence is critical, and it should be extended up to 24-25 years of age – the time when skeleton maturation is reached. The peak bone mass attained by the time of skeleton maturation is the most important factor in bone mass condition in older ages; therefore, deficient calcium intake during the period of active growth could not only condition the predicted final height, but would also be a risk factor for osteoporosis and osteoporotic fractures in adult life [1-4].

The recommended daily intake for calcium in people aged 9-18 is 1300 mg per day. Additionally, at least 60% of daily dietary calcium should be acquired through milk and derivatives, given its higher bioavailability in those forms [5, 6]. Therefore, dairy products should provide at least 780 mg of calcium on a daily basis during that age period (9-18 years), which would correspond with the intake of three servings of dairy products (equivalent dairy products with an estimated 250-300 mg calcium contribution) that is recommended by the food pyramid [7].

Food consumption surveys show how milk and its derivatives intake demonstrates a decreasing trend along with age, which could condition the maximum bone mineral content that is presumably reached within the third decade of life [8-13]. This potential nutritional impairment justifies the interest in evaluating milk and its derivatives intake in those sectors of the population whose bone mineralization is still in a critical, yet malleable situation, as it is in schoolchildren and adolescents.

The aim of the present chapter is to make a descriptive study of milk and its derivatives intake in a population of schoolchildren and adolescents, and to subsequently analyze its nutritional contribution to the diet of this population.

MATERIAL AND METHODS

A nutritional survey was carried out in a sample of 353 primary education students (schoolchildren group), aged 9 to 12, and in 406 secondary education students (adolescents group) aged 13 to 16, from four public school centers in the city of Pamplona (Navarre, Spain) from January-June, 2013.

Surveys were conducted by means of face-to-face interviews with students in the last course of their degree in human nutrition and dietetics at the University of Navarre.

The method they used was the registration of food intake during three consecutive academic days. Every student was asked about their food intake within the previous three consecutive days for every meal (breakfast, mid-morning snack, lunch, afternoon snack, and dinner).

With respect to dairy product intake, a serving of dairy was defined as the following amounts of dairy products: a glass of milk (250 ml), two yogurts (250 g), semi-mature cheese (60 g), fresh cheese (120 g), smoothies (250 ml), junket (150 g), custard-pudding (250 ml), and ice cream (200 ml). The calculation of the size of the portions corresponding to the different food groups was made using a photographic notebook from the *Institut Scientifique et Technique de la Nutrition et de l´Alimentation* (París, 2002) [14] to estimate and monitor the consistency of portion sizes.

Calorie and macronutrient (proteins, carbohydrates, total fat, saturated fatty acids (SFA), monounsaturated fatty acids (MUFA) and polyunsaturated fatty acids (PUFA), total fiber and cholesterol), mineral (calcium, iron, iodine, magnesium, zinc, selenium, and phosphorus), and vitamin (thiamine, riboflavin, niacin, vitamin B6, folates, vitamin B12, vitamin C, vitamin A, vitamin D, and vitamin E) intake was calculated individually using the Nutrition Calculation Program CESNID 1.0® (Centro de Enseñanza Superior de Nutrición y Dietética. Universidad de Barcelona) [15]. The updated charts of the National Academy of Sciences [16] were used as reference values for the daily recommended intake (dietary reference intake) of minerals and vitamins.

The results are displayed as means (m) and percentages (%) with corresponding standard deviations (SD) or confidence intervals (95% CI). Statistical analysis (Student's T, comparison of proportions) was conducted using the program SPSS version 20.0 (Chicago, Illinois, USA). Statistical significance was assumed when the p value<0.05.

RESULTS

Characteristics of the Sample

The group of primary education students was composed of 188 males (53.3%) and 165 females (46.7%); the average age was 10.51 (CI 95%: 10.3-10.7). The group of secondary education students consisted of 194 males (47.8%) and 212 females (52.2%); the average age was 14.6 (CI 95%: 14.5-14.7).

Consumption Frequencies

Table 1 shows the consumption frequencies of milk and its derivatives in the different daily meals for the entire sample. There were no statistically significant differences between the age groups.

Table 1. Consumption frequencies (%) for milk and other dairy products from different meals

Meals	Milk (%)	Yogurt (%)	Cheese (%)	Other Dairy (%)
Breakfast	88.3	3.5	2.2	0.1
Mid-morning snack	5.3	4.0	8.3	0.2
Lunch	4.4	28.4	4.4	5.2
Mid-afternoon snack	9.4	8.7	3.4	2.0
Dinner	16.0	29.8	18.3	5.5

Dairy product intake was reported by 94% of the respondents during breakfast, 69.3% for dinner, 42.1% for lunch, 23.3% for the afternoon snack, and 16.4% for their mid-morning snack. Milk intake was mainly associated with breakfast (88.3%), yogurt consumption in lunch (28.4%) and/or dinner (29.8%), and cheese intake was quite frequent during dinner (18.3%).

Milk and Other Dairy Product Intake

Table 2 shows and compares the average values of daily milk intake and its derivatives in the study groups by age and sex. The consumption of milk, yogurt, other dairy products, and total dairy products was significantly higher (p< 0.05) in the adolescent group.

The consumption of yogurt was significantly higher (p< 0.05) in males within the schoolchildren group. The intake of total dairy products was significantly higher (p<0.05) in males within both groups.

All respondents within the schoolchildren group reported drinking whole milk, whereas 21.7% of adolescents consumed skim or semi-skim milk (p<0.05). In the same way, 82.8% and 85.3% of the intake of yogurt in schoolchildren and adolescents was in the form of flavored whole milk yogurt, respectively (n.s.). Within the schoolchildren group, 82.2% of cheese intake was in the form of mature cheese and 17.8% was as fresh cheese, whereas within the adolescents group, mature cheese intake was 59.7% and fresh cheese was 40.3%, respectively (p<0.05).

Table 2. Average daily intake of milk (ml) and other daily products (g) in study groups by age and sex

Age groups (years)	Milk (ml)	Yogurt (g)	Cheese (g)	Other Dairy (g)	Total Dairy (g)
9 to 12					
Boys	277.2	97.5	15.4	23.7	413.8
Girls	264.3	62.5	18.4	20.4	365.6
Total	266.5*	80.1*	16.9	20.8*	384.3*
13 to 16					
Boys	308.5	103.2	29.5	47.2	488.4
Girls	294.7	91.9	22.8	43.6	453.0
Total	305.1*	96.4*	26.8	45.4*	473.7*

(*) p<0.05 among groups of age.

In terms of the consumption of other dairy products, within the schoolchildren, 50.5% of the intake was in the form of custard, whereas within adolescents, 44.3% of the intake was as pudding. From the total dairy product intake, skim milk represented 1% and 14.8% (p<0.05) in schoolchildren and adolescents, respectively.

Table 3 exposes and compares the percentage contribution of milk and derivatives to total dairy product intake, as well as the average values for the number of dairy servings by age group. From the total amount of dairy product intake, milk and yogurts represented 87.1%, showing no statistically significant differences among age groups and sexes. The mean value for the number of servings consumed by the entire group of surveyed students was 2 servings per day, and was significantly higher (p<0.05) in the adolescent group.

Calorie and Nutrient Intake

Table 4 displays and compares the average values for calorie, macronutrient, cholesterol, mineral, and vitamin intake provided by milk and derivatives by age groups. The contribution of calories, as well as some macronutrients (proteins and carbohydrates), minerals (calcium, iodine, magnesium, sodium and potassium), and vitamins (folates and vitamin A) were significantly higher (p<0.05) in the adolescent group.

Percentage Contribution of Food Groups

Table 5 shows and compares the percentage values for nutrients provided by milk and derivatives in relation to the total daily intake (%TI), as well as in relation to the established recommendation (%DRIs). In both groups, milk and its derivatives mainly contributed to the total daily intake of calories (18.1%), proteins (21.5%), total fat (26.4%), SFA (36.7%) and cholesterol (20%). Milk and its derivatives also contributed to minerals: calcium (72.1%), iodine (51.2%), phosphorous (36.4%), potassium (28.5%), magnesium (23.36%), and zinc (17.7%) and vitamins: vitamin A (47.8%), riboflavin (40%) and vitamin B12 (42%). In the same way, milk and its derivatives contributed largely to the dietary reference intake of proteins (21.5%) and carbohydrates (25%), as well as minerals: calcium (48.1%), phosphorous (40.7%), iodine (30.9%), zinc (24.7%), magnesium (19.6%), and sodium (21,3%) and vitamins: riboflavin (78.8%), vitamin B12 (65%), vitamin A (27.8%), niacin (29.9%), and pyridoxine (18.3%).

Table 3. Percentage contribution (%) to the total dairy product intake from milk and its derivatives and average values for the number of portions by age groups

Age groups (years)	Milk (%)	Yogurt (%)	Cheese (%)	Other Dairy (%)	Portions (number)
9 to 12	69.3	20.8	4.4	5.5	1.75
13 to 16	64.4	20.4	5.7	9.5	2.22*
Total	66.6	20.5	5.2	7.8	2.00

(*) $p < 0.05$ among age groups.

Table 4. Average calorie and nutrient intake per day from milk and dairy products in different age groups

Groups of age (years)	9 to 12 Mean (SD)	13 to 16 Mean (SD)
Energy (Kcal)	349 (105.9)	410 (124.4)*
Proteins (g)	18.3 (3.8)	22.6 (4.9)*
Carbohydrates (g)	28.2 (5.4)	37.4 (7.1)*
Fat (g)	18.1 (4.9)	18.9 (4.8)
SFA (g)	10.6 (2.5)	11.0 (2.7)
MUFA(g)	5.0 (1.6)	5.2 (1.7)
PUFA (g)	1.3 (0.2)	1.4 (0.3)
Cholesterol(mg)	58.2 (17.4)	60.8 (18.0)
Calcium (mg)	574 (109.6)	675 (128.2)*
Iron (mg)	0.44 (0.13)	0.51 (0.16)
Iodine (mg)	35.7 (9.7)	47.6 (13.0)*
Magnesium (mg)	49.9 (13.1)	70.3 (18.6)*
Zinc (mg)	2.0 (0.4)	2.4 (0.5)
Selenium (µg)	5.5 (1.5)	7.0 (2.1)
Sodium (mg)	291 (51.2)	346 (65.6)*
Potassium (mg)	670 (117.2)	797 (141.1)*
Phosphorous (mg)	462 (84.5)	555 (101.6)*
Thiamin (mg)	0.15 (0.05)	0.17 (0.05)
Riboflavin (mg)	0.74 (0.2)	0.86 (0.23)
Niacin (mg)	3.5 (0.6)	4.5 (0.87)
Pyridoxine (mg)	0.19 (0.06)	0.22 (0.07)
Folates (µg)	28.3 (12.5)	34.4 (15.2)*
B12 (mg)	1.2 (0.5)	1.5 (0,6)
Vit. C (mg)	4.6 (2.8)	5.5 (3.4)
Vit. A (µg)	186 (81.9)	194 (85.4)*
Vit. D (UI)	88.5 (56.0)	95.0 (61.2)
Vit. E (mg)	0.43 (0.19)	0.46 (0.2)

Table 5. Contribution (%) of milk and its derivatives to total intake of energy and nutrients (%TI) in relation to the dietary reference intakes (%DRIs)

Age groups (years)	9 to12		13 to 16	
	(%TI)	(%DRIs)	(%TI)	(%DRIs)
Calories	18.5	ND	17.7	ND
Proteins	19.7	54.3	23.2	45.5
Carbohydrates	9.0	21.8	15.6	28.2
Total fat	36.9	ND	15.8	ND
SFA	47.5	ND	25.8	ND
MUFA	32.4	ND	10.9	ND
PUFA	23.8	ND	5.3	ND
Cholesterol	20.2	ND	19.8	ND
Calcium (mg)	71.8	44.7	72.3	51.4
Iron (mg)	2.7	5.6	8.3	4.0
Iodine (mg)	43.7	30.2	58.7	31.5
Magnesium (mg)	20.9	21.0	25.6	18.1
Zinc (mg)	19.8	25.1	15.5	24.2
Selenium (µg)	5.1	14.1	8.3	12.5
Sodium (mg)	11.7	19.6	22.0	22.9
Potassium (mg)	22.8	15.0	34.2	16.7
Phosphorous (mg)	35.0	37.4	37.7	43.9
Thiamin (mg)	11.2	16.7	16.9	15.5
Riboflavin (mg)	41.3	82.8	37.8	74.8
Niacin (mg)	10.3	30.0	11.9	29.7
Pyridoxine (mg)	9.9	19.0	16.0	17.6
Folates (µg)	9.4	9.5	18.0	8.5
B12 (mg)	38.3	69.5	45.6	60.4
Vit. C (mg)	9.4	10.4	15.3	7.8
Vit. A (µg)	47.6	31.4	48.0	24.1
Vit. D (UI)	7.2	3.2	8.0	3.8
Vit. E (mg)	11.4	4.0	7.5	3.1

DISCUSSION

Nutritional surveys based on recall are an optimal and frequently used tool in cross-sectional studies for descriptive purposes, just as it occurs in this chapter [17]. In this case, it is remarkable how interviews were carried out by sufficiently qualified personnel; additionally, a photographic notebook with portion and serving size examples was used to help the respondents specify the quantity and/or size of the corresponding servings from the previous 3 days as accurately as possible. In this way, respondents were able to identify portions and/or serving sizes, so interviewers could estimate the intake [14]. However, this chapter has several methodological limitations, because sociological variables, such as socioeconomic status, educational level, and/or life style, etc. were not registered, and they could condition, to some extent, the dietary intake.

When analyzing the consumption frequencies for different types of dairy products, it is worth nothing that almost every respondent consumed dairy products throughout the day, whole milk being a basic food for breakfast, while plain or flavored yogurt (and full-fat yogurt) was a relatively frequent food for lunch and/or dinner. The intake of other dairy products, including different kinds of cheese, was, in comparison, less frequent. These registered consumption frequencies could explain how the total number of dairy servings in both age groups, even though it was significantly higher in adolescents, did not reach the three recommended daily servings. Moreover, as a consequence of this deficient ingestion of dairy products, the intake of dietary calcium from milk and its derivatives barely reached 48% of the dietary reference intake for the age groups analyzed, even though it represented 72% of the daily dietary calcium. It should be mentioned how a maintained dairy product intake below the established recommendations implies the need to consume dietary and/or pharmacological calcium supplements, since there would not be adequate assurance of normal bone apposition.

The variety of dairy products consumed by these young students has a number of peculiarities that should be further analyzed. When studying the contribution of milk and derivatives to the daily nutrient intake within these analyzed populations, we confirmed how, despite the deficient intake of dairy servings with respect to the established recommendations, this food group still constituted the main dietary source of calcium, iodine, magnesium, and phosphorous, as well as riboflavin, vitamin B12, and vitamin A; they also contributed substantially to the daily intake of calories, proteins, potassium, and zinc. In the same way, the recorded dairy product consumption largely contributed to fulfill the recommended dietary allowance for proteins and carbohydrates, as well as different minerals (calcium, phosphorous, iodine, zinc, magnesium, and sodium) and vitamins (riboflavin, vitamin B12, vitamin A, niacin, and pyridoxine) [18-21]. Nevertheless, it should be emphasized that dietary milk calcium in both groups barely reached 48% of the daily dietary reference intake for these age groups, as had been reported by authors in our cultural-geographic environment [19-24], being far below the percentage of daily dietary calcium that should be provided by milk and its derivatives in order to obtain adequate bone mass.

However, although the daily intake of dairy products should be increased to make up for the deficient calcium intake that has been observed in schoolchildren and adolescents, milk intake and its derivatives also contributed substantially to the intake of total fat, SFA, and cholesterol. These could be noticeably reduced by consuming low-fat and/or modified fatty acid composition dairy products [23]. The consumption of low-fat products in schoolchildren is virtually non-existent and represents scarcely 15% of the total dairy product ingestion. Therefore, it should be required to recommend the daily consumption of skim or low-fat dairy products (milk and yogurts) to these students, as well as the different varieties of fresh cheese available in the market (Burgos cheese, petit Suisse, cottage, mozzarella, etc.). In this way, the content of minerals and vitamins would increase without increasing the calorie, SFA, and cholesterol intake. Likewise, the avoidance of milk derivatives, with their high content of carbohydrates and cholesterol (custard, pudding, etc.), should be promoted.

In conclusion, the intake of milk and its derivatives in the child and juvenile population is inappropriate. Consequently, the need to undertake a massive public enlightenment campaign to increase awareness among families in terms of the nutritional importance of this food group should be seriously considered. Moreover, they should be advised on dietary alternatives that are available in current markets, such as low-fat and high nutritive value (minerals and vitamins) dairy products, which could noticeably contribute to the appropriate dietary calcium intake required to achieve an optimal peak of bone mass, as well as other nutrients that have additional beneficial effects for human health.

REFERENCES

[1]   Borrajo E, Gutierez-Macias A, Gutierrez-Sánchez E. Osteoporosis. In Dieguez C., Iturriaga R. (ed): "Metabolismo fosfocálcico," Madrid: McGraw-Hill, pp 113-131, 2003.

[2]   Lanou AJ, Berkow SE, Barnard ND. Calcium, dairy products, and bone health in children and young adults: a reevaluation of the evidence. *Pediatrics* 2005; 115:736-743.

[3]   Fiorito LM, Mitchell DC, Smiciklas-Wright H, Birch LL. Girls' calcium intake is associated with bone mineral content during middle childhood. *J Nutr.* 2006; 136:1281-1286.

[4]   Huth PJ, DiRienzo DB, Miller GD. Major scientific advances with dairy foods in nutrition and health. *J Dairy Sci* 2006; 89:1207-1221.

[5]   Infante D, Tormo R. Risk of inadequate bone mineralization in diseases involving long-term suppression of dairy products. *J Pediatr Gastroenterol Nutr* 2000; 30:310-313.

[6]   Greer FR, Krebs NF. American Academy of Pediatrics Committee on Nutrition: Optimizing bone health and calcium intakes of infants, children, and adolescents. *Pediatrics* 2006; 117:578-585.

[7]   Fulgoni VL 3rd, Huth PJ, DiRienzo DB, Miller GD. Determination of the optimal number of dairy servings to ensure a low prevalence of inadequate calcium intake in Americans. *J Am Coll Nutr* 2004; 23:651-659.

[8]   Durá Travé T. Energy and nutrient intake in compulsory high school students. *An Esp Pediatr* 2001; 54:547-54.

[9]   Rajeshwari R, Nicklas TA, Yang SJ, Berenson GS. Longitudinal changes in intake and food sources of calcium from childhood to young adulthood: the Bogalusa Heart Study. *J Am Coll Nutr* 2004; 23:341-350.

[10]   Fiorito LM, Mitchell DC, Smiciklas-Wright H, Birch LL. Dairy and dairy-related nutrient intake during middle childhood. *J Am Diet Assoc* 2006; 106:534-542.

[11]   Durá-Travé T. Intake of milk and dairy products in a college population. *Nutr Hosp* 2008; 23:91-96.

[12]   Baird DL, Syrette J, Hendrie GA, Riley MD, Bowen J, Noakes M. Dairy food intake of Australian children and adolescents 2-16 years of age: 2007 Australian National Children's Nutrition and Physical Activity Survey. *Public Health Nutr* 2012; 15:2060-2073.

[13]   Dror DK, Allen LH. Dairy product intake in children and adolescents in developed countries: trends, nutritional contribution, and a review of association with health outcomes. *Nutr Rev* 2014; 72: 68-81.

[14]   SU.VI.MAX. Portions alimentaires. Manuel photos pour l'estimation des quantite´s. Paris: Polytechnica, 2002.

[15]   Centre d'Ensenyament Superior de Nutríció i Dietètica. Programa de cálculo nutricional CESNID 1.0 (Cd-rom). Barcelona: McGraw-Hill, 2003.

[16]   Dietary References Intakes: Macronutrients, Elements and vitamins. Food and Nutrition Board, Institute of Medicine, National Academy of

Sciences, 2004. Available at URL: http://www.nap.edu25 (accessed on 26 August 2013).

[17] Martínez MA, Alonso A, Egües N.: Sistemas de evaluación del consumo de alimentos. In Muñoz M., Aranceta J., García-Jalón I. (ed.): "Nutrición aplicada y dietoterapia". Pamplona: EUNSA, pp. 67-82, 2004.

[18] Gaucheron F. Milk and dairy products: A unique micronutrient combination. *J Am Col. Nutr* 2011; 30: 400S-409S.

[19] Drewnowski A. The contribution of milk and milk products to micronutrient density and affordability of the U.S. diet. *J Am Coll Nutr* 30(5 Suppl. 1): 422S-428S, 2011.

[20] Vissers PA, Streppel MT, Feskens EJ, de Groot LC. The contribution of dairy products to micronutrient intake in the Netherlands. *J Am Coll Nutr* 2011; 30 (Suppl. 1): 415S-421S.

[21] Coudray B. The contribution of dairy products to micronutrient intakes in France. *J Am Coll Nutr* 2011; 30(5 Suppl. 1):410S-414S.

[22] Suárez Cortina L, Moreno Villares JM, Martínez Suárez V, Aranceta Bartrina J, Dalmau Serra J, Gil Hernández A, et al. Calcium intake and bone mineral density in a group of Spanish school-children. *An Pediatr (Barc)* 2001; 74: 3-9.

[23] Ortega RM, López-Sobaler AM, Jiménez Ortega AI, Navia Lombán B, Ruiz-Roso Calvo de Mora B, Rodríguez-Rodríguez E, et al. Food sources and average intake of calcium in a representative sample of Spanish schoolchildren. *Nutr Hosp* 2012; 27: 715-23.

[24] Spence L. A., Cifelli C. J., Miller G. D.: The Role of Dairy Products in Healthy Weight and Body Composition in Children and Adolescents. *Curr Nutr Food Sci* 2011; 7: 40-49.

In: Focus on Nutrition …
Editor: Teodoro Durá-Travé

ISBN: 978-1-63463-223-2
© 2015 Nova Science Publishers, Inc.

Chapter 8

NUTRITIONAL ANALYSIS OF BREAKFAST ON RISING AND MID-MORNING SNACK IN AN UNDERGRADUATE POPULATION

Teodoro Durá-Travé[1,2], Fidel Gallinas-Victoriano[2], Beatriz Durá-Gúrpide[1], Carlos Andrés-Sesma[2] and Marta Martínez-Merino[2]

[1]Department of Pediatrics, Faculty of Medicine,
University of Navarra, Pamplona, Spain
[2]Department of Pediatrics, Navarra Hospital Complex,
Pamplona, Spain

ABSTRACT

Objective: To carry out a descriptive study on the breakfast model in an undergraduate population and to analyze the energy and nutrients provided, in connection with established nutritional requirements.

Material and Methods: Registry of food intake for breakfast (on rising and as a mid-morning snack) on a school day in a sample of 740 undergraduate students (286 men and 454 women) with ages ranging from 19-24. Sex, age, weight, height, body mass index, and type of residence were collected from each interviewed subject. The percentage intake of nutrients has been calculated in relation to established dietary recommendations (%DRIs).

Results: 93.2% had breakfast upon rising and 83.8% had a daily mid-morning snack; 53.5% performed both intakes. The most common foods were dairy products (92.6%), cereals (58.8%), and industrial pastries (57.9%) at breakfast, while cereals (46.6%), fruits (40.7%), and sausages (34.9%) were consumed at mid-morning. The %DRIs of the calorie intake was 24.4% in males and 24.6% in females (n.s.). The %DRIs of cholesterol intake was 38.2% in males and 23.9% in females (p<0.05). The %DRIs for minerals and vitamins was greater (p < 0.05) for early breakfasts.

Conclusions: This breakfast model differs from the prototype of a healthy diet due to an excessive consumption of industrial pastries (early breakfast), meat, and derivatives (snack). Half of the interviewee did not participate in a mid-morning snack and the morning caloric intake was below the recommended level.

INTRODUCTION

Breakfast is widely known as one of the most important daily dietary intakes, and, in fact, a balanced daily breakfast has been associated with an optimal nutrient intake throughout the day and better physical and intellectual performance [1-5]; however, it is often ignored, forgotten, or poorly done [6,7]. An adequate breakfast reinforces, from the early morning, the commitment to a healthy way of life, and, whenever breakfast is absent, it complicates the achievement of daily dietary recommendations, particularly in terms of minerals and vitamins [8-11]; cognitive functions, and consequently academic performance, may be negatively affected.

In order to ensure a nutritional balance, it is essential that your diet contains a variety of different foods and, obviously, the first daily intake – breakfast – should not be an exception to this rule. Breakfast should contribute one quarter of the total daily caloric needs, and the composition of a balanced breakfast should include food from at least three of the basic groups: dairy products, cereals, and fruits. The diversification of foods should let breakfast be a healthy and palatable meal, in addition to providing its nutritional components [12-14].

There is a deep-rooted tradition, in our geographical area, of having a first intake – breakfast – before leaving home. After that, a second snack at mid-morning that would complement the morning intake and allows for the delaying of the main midday intake – lunch [6, 15, 16]. Therefore, in this geographical and cultural area, a distinction between a first (breakfast itself) and a second morning meal (usually a mid-morning snack or brunch) should be made.

The purpose of this chapter is to describe the characteristics of the breakfast model in an undergraduate population, as well as to analyze the energy and nutrient intake of these students in relation to the established nutritional requirements.

MATERIAL AND METHODS

A nutritional survey was distributed and subsequently fulfilled in a random sample of 740 undergraduate students in different faculties and schools within the university campus of the *University of Navarra* at Pamplona (Architecture, Sciences, Law, Nursing, Economics, Pharmacy, Medicine, and Literature) in the second semester of the 2011/2012 academic year. Surveys were conducted by students of the Degree in Human Nutrition and Dietetics by means of personal interviews. Every respondent was asked in detail about their intake during the morning of a school day (breakfast and/or mid-morning snack). Information on sex, age, anthropometric variables (weight, height, and body mass index), and type of accommodation (student apartment, home stay, or student residence) was also collected.

Body mass index (BMI) was calculated according to the following formula: Weight (kg)/height^2 (m). Four groups were defined depending on the BMI value: undernourishment (BMI<18.5), normality (18.5-24.99), overweight (25-29.99), and obesity (>30).

The food was divided into different groups:

1. Milk and derivatives (dairy products)
2. Cereals and derivatives (bread/toast, breakfast cereals, etc.)
3. Sweets, industrial pastries, and bakery products (chocolate, jam, biscuits, croissants, sponge cake, etc.)
4. Fruits and juices
5. Fat and oil (butter, margarine, olive oil, etc.)
6. Meat and derivatives
7. Eggs and derivatives
8. Vegetables and tubers (potatoes)
9. Fish

Energy and macronutrients intake (proteins, carbohydrates, total fat, saturated fatty acids (SFA), monounsaturated fatty acids (MUFA), polyunsaturated fatty acids (PUFA), cholesterol, and total fiber) minerals (calcium, iron, iodine, magnesium, zinc, selenium, and phosphate), and vitamins (thiamine, riboflavin, niacin, vitamin B6, folate, vitamin B12, vitamin C, vitamin A, vitamin D, and vitamin E) were calculated using the nutrition calculation software CESNID 1.0® (Centro de Enseñanza Superior de Nutrición y Dietética. Universidad de Barcelona) [17]. The revised tables of the *National Academy of Sciences* [18] were applied as reference values for the dietary reference intakes (DRIs) of minerals and vitamins.

The results are displayed as means (M) and percentages (%) with corresponding standard deviations (SD) or 95% confidence intervals (95% CI). A statistical analysis (Student's t, Chi square tests and comparison of proportions) was done using the *Statistical Packages for the Social Sciences* (SPSS) version 20.0 software (Chicago, Illinois, EE.UU.). The statistical significance was assumed when the *p* value <0.05.

RESULTS

Characteristics of the Sample

The sample consisted of 740 undergraduate students (286 males and 454 females). The age of the respondents ranged from 18 to 25, with an average of 20.47±1.67 years (CI 95%: 20.35-20.59). Table 1 set out the distribution of the surveyed students by sex according to age, type of accommodation, and nutritional status. There were no significant differences among the age groups and types of accommodation between sexes. However, the percentage values of overweight/obesity in males (20.8%) were significantly higher (p<0.05) than in females (6.7%).

BMI (kg/m^2) for males was 23.4 (CI 95%: 23.1-23.7), significantly higher (p<0.05) than that of females (21.1), (CI 95%: 20.8-21.4).

The daily consumption of breakfast and mid-morning snacks was referred to by 98.6% (n=730, 279 males and 451 females) and 54.2% (n=401, 149 males and 252 females) of the respondents, respectively. Consuming both meals was claimed by 53.5% (n=396, 149 males and 252 females).

Table 1. Distribution of undergraduate students by sex, age, anthropometric data and nutritional status

	Males n (%)	Females n (%)	Total n (%)
Age group			
18-19 years	94 (32.9)	137 (30.2)	231 (31.2)
20-21 years	121 (42.3)	216 (47.5)	337 (45.5)
22-23 years	57 (19.9)	78 (17.2)	135 (18.3)
24-25 years	14 (4.9)	23 (5.1)	37 (5.0)
Place of residence			
Student apartment	118 (41.2)	194 (42.7)	312 (42.2)
Home stay	98 (34.3)	161 (35.5)	259 (35.0)
Student Residence	70 (24.5)	99 (21.8)	169 (22.8)
Nutritional status*			
Undernourishment	7 (2.5)	41 (9.2)	48 (6.6)
Normality	218 (76.7)	376 (84.1)	594 (81.3)
Overweight	49 (17.3)	27 (6.0)	76 (10.4)
Obesity	10 (3.5)	3 (0.7)	13 (1.8)

(*) $p < 0.05$.

Consumption Frequencies

Table 2 outlines and compares the consumption frequencies of the different food groups in breakfast and mid-morning snacks among the respondents. As for breakfast, milk and derivatives (92.6%), cereals and derivatives (58.8%), sweets, industrial pastries, and bakery products (57.9%) and, to a lesser extent, fruits and natural juices (36.4%) and fat and oil (20.4%) were the food groups that showed the highest frequency. In addition, 47.6% of the respondents added sugar, coffee, or cocoa powder to milk. The most common type of breakfast (26.4% of the surveyed students) consisted of a glass of whole milk (with/without the addition of sugar, coffee, or cocoa powder) plus cookies or industrial pastries. In terms of the mid-morning snack, cereals and derivatives (46.6%), fruits or natural juices (40.7%), meat and derivatives (34.9%), and, to a lesser extent, milk and derivatives (28.9%) and sweets, pastries and bakery products (19.2%), were the food groups with more frequent consumption. Only 22.7% referred to the ingestion of one piece of fruit and 8.2% a glass of milk. There were no statistically significant differences between sexes.

Table 2. Daily consumption frequencies (%) for the different food groups in breakfast and mid-morning snacks

Food group	Breakfast %	Mid-morning snack %
Milk and derivatives*	92.6	28.9
Whole milk	69.6	15.7
Semi skimmed/skimmed milk	20.4	0.2
Yoghurt	4.7	4.5
Cheese	3.2	8.5
Cereals and derivatives*	58.8	46.6
Bread/toast	36.1	40.6
Breakfast cereals	22.7	6.0
Sweets, pastries, and bakery goods*	57.9	19.2
Cookies	22.6	6.5
Pastries	19.2	9.3
Jam	13.6	0.2
Other (chocolate, cakes, etc.)	1.5	3.2
Fruits and natural juices	36.4	40.7
Fruits	16.6	35.0
Juices*	26.7	5.7
Fat and oil*	20.4	2.0
Oil	11.1	0.5
Butter	9.3	1.5
Meat and derivatives*	8.4	34.9
Eggs and derivatives*	1.4	12.7
Vegetables and tubers		17.5
Tomatoes	---	6.0
Potatoes*		11.5
Fish	---	0.4

(*) $p < 0.05$.

The intake of milk and derivatives, at the expense of the different varieties of milk (whole or skimmed milk), as well as sweets, pastries, or bakery goods, natural juices, and fat and oil was significantly higher ($p < 0.05$) in breakfast, whereas the intake of meat and derivatives, eggs and derivatives, and tubers (potatoes) was significantly higher ($p < 0.05$) in mid-morning snacks.

Nutrient and Calorie Intake

Table 3 presents and compares the average values of nutrient and calorie intake in breakfast and mid-morning snacks in both sexes. The intake of calories and nutrients (proteins, carbohydrates, total fat, SFA, MUFA, PUFA, fiber, and cholesterol), as well as different minerals (calcium, iron, iodine, and phosphorus), and vitamins (thiamine, riboflavin, niacin, folate, and vitamins B_{12}, A, D, and E) in breakfast was significantly higher ($p<0.05$) in males. In the same way, the intake of calories and nutrients (proteins, carbohydrates, total fat, SFA, MUFA, PUFA, fiber, and cholesterol) and different minerals (calcium, iron, iodine, and phosphorus), and vitamins (thiamine, riboflavin, niacin, folate and vitamins B_{12}, A, D, and E) in mid-morning snacks was significantly higher ($p<0.05$) in males.

The comparison of total caloric and nutrient intake in breakfast and in mid-morning snacks reveals that calorie, macronutrient (except for cholesterol), mineral, and vitamin intake in breakfast was significantly higher ($p<0.05$).

Table 3. Intake of macronutrients, minerals and vitamins for both sexes in breakfast and mid-morning snack. (M±DS)

Nutrients	Breakfast		Mid-morning snack	
	Males (n=279)	Females (n=451)	Males (n=149)	Females (n=252)
Kcal	432.2±196.4*	333.6±136.9	276.6±163.2*	206.7±143.4
Proteins (g)	13.6±7.0*	10.6±4.0	10.6±8.7*	7.3±6.8
Carbohydrates (g)	56.0±27.0*	44.4±18.2	34.8±21.3*	28.2±17.0
Total fat(g)	16.4±9.7*	11.9±7.9	9.9±7.5*	6.6±5.1
SFA (g)	7.9±4.6*	5.8±4.0	4.0±3.5*	2.7±2.1
MUFA (g)	5.5±3.6*	4.1±3.0	3.5±2.6*	2.3±1.9
PUFA (g)	1.5±1.3*	1.1±0.9	1.2±1.1*	8.0±0.7
Total fiber (g)	3.0±2.0*	2.6±1.9	2.5±1.6	2.2±1.6
Cholesterol (mg)	61.9±48.2*	37.6±29.1	52.7±39.9*	34.2±27.2
Calcium (mg)	312.7±103.3*	270.7±98.9	105.2±96.5*	84.7±69.4
Iron (mg)	3.5±2.8*	2.7±2.3	1.9±1.3*	1.5±1.1
Iodine (µg)	23.0±9.2*	20.4±8.2	8.6±6.2*	6.6±5.0
Magnesium (mg)	52.2±23.2	48.8±24.4	27.0±16.4*	22.1±14.5
Zinc (mg)	1.6±0.7	1.5±1.1	1.1±0.7*	0.8±0.6
Selenium (µg)	16.3±10.7	15.6±11.6	14.7±11.2*	9.7±8.8

Table 3. (Continued)

Nutrients	Breakfast		Mid-morning snack	
	Males (n=279)	Females (n=451)	Males (n=149)	Females (n=252)
Phosphorus (mg)	294.4±102.9*	240.3±83.2	161.2±99.1*	120.7±77.4
Thiamine (mg)	0.47±0.31*	0.37±0.31	0.22±0.21*	0.17±0.16
Riboflavin (mg)	0.72±0.51*	0.62±0.45	0.21±0.17	0.18±0.15
Niacin (mg)	6.6±5.3*	5.3±4.2	3.9±3.1	2.9±2.1
Vitamin B_6(mg)	0.57±1.26	0.54±1.18	0.19±0.22	0.16±0.14
Folate (µg)	66.3±40.2*	52.3±38.6	24.1±18.3	22.2±15.7
VitaminB_{12}(mg)	0.93±0.90*	0.72±0.36	0.39±0.31*	0.27±0.33
Vitamin C(mg)	38.8±22.3	34.0±22.2	12.0±9.7	13.0±9.2
Vitamin A (µg)	165.2±91.2*	123.0±71.0	84.0±71.7	74.5±61.9
Vitamin D (µg)	0.92±1.12*	0.64±0.91	0.21±0.42	0.11±0.28
Vitamin E (mg)	0.92±0.78*	0.67±0.54	0.58±0.59	0.50±0.47

(*) $p < 0.05$ among sexes.

Percentages of Dietary Reference Intakes (%Rdis)

In terms of breakfast, the average value for caloric intake in comparison to reference intake (%RDIs) was 14.9% in males and 15.2% in females (NS); for mid-morning snacks, the average value in males was 9.5%, and 9.4% in females (NS). The average values of %IR for total calorie intake (breakfast and mid-morning snack) was 24.4% in males and 24.6% in females (NS).

In terms of breakfast, 20.6% of males and 12.5% of females (NS) overtook the average percent value for the upper limit of the daily reference intake of cholesterol (300 mg/day); this value was 17.6% in males and 11.4% in females for mid-morning snacks. For breakfast and mid-morning snacks, 38.2% of males and 23.9% of females ($p < 0.05$) overtook the average percent value for the upper limit of the daily reference intake of total cholesterol.

Table 4 shows and compares the %DRIs for the intake of minerals and vitamins in both sexes in relation to breakfast and mid-morning snacks. The %DRIs for minerals and vitamins was significantly higher ($p < 0.05$) in breakfast than in mid-morning snacks. There were no statistically significant differences in %DRIs according to sex in breakfast or mid-morning snacks, except in the case of iron intake.

Table 4. Percentage of reference intake (%DRIs) of minerals and vitamins for both sexes in breakfast and mid-morning snack

Nutrients	Breakfast %DRIs		Mid-morning snack %DRIs		Total %DRIs	
	Males	Females	Males	Females	Males	Females
Calcium (mg)	31.3	27.1	10.5	8.5	41.8	35.6
Iron (mg)	43.8*	15.0	23.8*	8.3	67.6*	23.3
Iodine (µg)	15.3	13.6	5.7	4.4	21.0	18.3
Magnesium (mg)	13.1	15.7	6.8	7.1	19.9	22.8
Zinc (mg)	14.5	18.8	10.0	10.0	24.5	28.8
Selenium (µg)	29.6	28.4	26.7	17.6	56.3	46.0
Phosphorus (mg)	42.1	34.3	23.0	17.2	65.1	51.5
Thiamine (mg)	39.2	33.6	18.3	15.5	57.5	49.1
Riboflavin(mg)	55.4	56.4	16.2	16.4	71.6	72.8
Niacin (mg)	41.3	37.9	24.4	20.7	65.7	58.6
Vitamin B_6(mg)	43.8	41.5	14.6	12.3	58.4	53.8
Folate (µg)	16.6	13.1	6.0	5.6	22.6	18.7
Vitamin B_{12}(mg)	38.8	30.0	16.3	11.3	55.1	41.3
Vitamin C(mg)	43.1	45.3	13.3	17.3	56.4	62.6
Vitamin A (µg)	18.4	17.6	9.3	10.6	27.7	28.2
Vitamin D (µg)	18.4	12.8	4.2	2.2	22.6	15.0
Vitamin E (mg)	6.1	4.5	3.9	3.3	10.0	7.8

(*) $p < 0.05$ among sexes.

Percentage Contribution of Food Groups

Table 5 exposes the percentage contribution of calorie and nutrient intake for the food groups with a higher frequency of consumption in breakfast. Three of the food groups (milk and derivatives, sweets, pastries and bakery products, and cereals and derivatives) account for 82.6% of the caloric intake. Milk and derivatives provide mostly proteins, total fat, SFA, MUFA, cholesterol, calcium, iodine, magnesium, zinc, phosphorus, riboflavin, vitamin $B_{12,}$ and vitamin A. Cereals and derivatives primarily provide proteins, carbohydrates, fiber, iron, zinc, selenium, thiamine, riboflavin, niacin, folate, vitamin B_6, vitamin A, and vitamin D. Sweets, pastries, and bakery products contribute carbohydrates, total fat, SFA, MUFA, PUFA, cholesterol, and vitamin E. Fruits and juices provide fiber, folate, vitamin C, and vitamin E. Finally, fat and oil mainly contribute PUFA.

Table 6 illustrates the percent contribution of calories and nutrients for the most frequent food groups consumed in mid-morning snacks. Three of them (cereals and derivatives, sweets, pastries and bakery products, and meat and derivatives) account for 62.7% of the total energy intake. Cereals and derivatives provide proteins, carbohydrates, fiber, iron, magnesium, selenium, thiamine, riboflavin, niacin, vitamin B_6, folate, and vitamin D, while sweets, pastries, and bakery products contribute mainly to total fat, SFA, MUFA and PUFA. The contribution of meat and derivatives is mainly in the form of proteins, total fat, SFA, MUFA, PUFA, cholesterol, zinc, thiamine, niacin, vitamin B12, and vitamin A. Milk and derivatives mainly contribute proteins, total fat, SFA, calcium, iodine, magnesium, zinc, phosphorus, riboflavin, vitamin B_{12}, and vitamin A. Fruits and juices are responsible for providing carbohydrates, fiber, magnesium, vitamin B_6, folate, vitamin C, and E. Finally, eggs mainly contain cholesterol, vitamin B_{12}, and vitamin D.

Table 5. Percent contribution (%) of the most frequently consumed food groups in terms of calorie and nutrient intake for breakfast

Nutrients	Food group				
	Milk	Cereals	Sweets	Fruits	Fat
Kilocalories	29.5	22.0	31.1	9.3	5.3
Proteins	51.0	22.9	13.6	4.2	---
Carbohydrates	17.2	31.1	36.6	14.9	---
Total fat	42.1	6.0	30.3	1.3	16.2
SFA	51.7	2.3	27.4	0.4	15.0
MUFA	35.2	6.6	30.8	0.9	21.8
PUFA	17.1	16.2	47.0	3.4	8.5
Fiber	---	44.6	26.0	29.4	---
Cholesterol	42.5	---	37.3	---	7.9
Calcium	79.0	8.8	8.5	3.3	0.07
Iron	5.7	66.7	18.0	5.7	0.3
Iodine	75.3	8.1	7.6	3.8	2.5
Magnesium	49.6	17.9	13.3	17.3	---
Zinc	52.4	21.9	11.2	6.3	---
Selenium	18.2	59.9	16.2	5.2	---
Phosphorus	66.6	13.6	12.2	4.5	0.13
Thiamin	19.0	57.1	9.5	11.9	---

Nutrients	Food group				
	Milk	Cereals	Sweets	Fruits	Fat
Riboflavin	51.6	39.1	6.3	3.1	---
Niacin	23.3	56.6	11.0	3.8	---
Vitamin B_6	19.0	64.3	4.8	11.9	---
Folate	15.5	51.5	9.4	22.8	---
Vitamin B_{12}	67.9	16.7	12.8	---	---
Vitamin C	6.4	21.7	1.0	70.8	---
Vitamin A	49.4	29.2	7.3	3.7	9.0
Vitamin D	6.6	85.5	5.3	---	1.3
Vitamin E	18.9	5.4	27.0	32.4	12.2

Table 6. Percent contribution (%) of the most frequently consumed food groups in terms of calorie and nutrient intake of mid-morning snacks

Nutrients	Food group					
	Milk	Cereals	Sweets	Fruits	Meat	Egg
Kilocalories	13.8	28.8	18.2	14.5	15.7	2.6
Proteins	25.5	25.5	7.2	3.5	29.8	5.4
Carbohydrates	7.2	42.3	17.1	22.8	3.0	---
Total fat	21.0	5.1	25.9	2.5	32.1	5.9
SFA	31.3	3.2	25.8	0.9	30.6	4.2
MUFA	16.2	3.4	25.9	2.4	37.9	6.9
PUFA	8.3	9.1	30.0	5.7	32.0	7.2
Fiber	---	37.2	9.3	48.5	---	---
Cholesterol	15.4	---	19.2	---	25.4	39.0
Calcium	67.3	13.1	7.6	7.0	1.9	1.9
Iron	3.7	46.3	11.0	16.3	16.8	4.2
Iodine	47.4	13.4	6.4	9.1	15.5	5.3
Magnesium	32.1	23.1	7.7	20.5	7.7	1.5
Zinc	21.8	17.3	6.4	8.2	34.5	7.3
Selenium	8.7	59.1	11.0	7.6	8.7	3.1
Phosphorus	40.3	18.0	8.1	6.2	16.5	5.8
Thiamin	18.2	31.8	9.1	13.6	27.2	---
Riboflavin	40.0	28.0	4.0	12.0	12.0	8.0
Niacin	13.8	35.9	7.7	4.6	28.2	3.3
Vitamin B_6	9.5	38.1	4.8	23.8	14.3	---
Folate	9.7	42.1	5.4	28.8	2.2	6.7
Vitamin B_{12}	37.5	10.0	7.5	---	25.0	20.0

Table 6. (Continued)

Nutrients	Food group					
	Milk	Cereals	Sweets	Fruits	Meat	Egg
Vitamin C	4.1	12.4	0.1	80.0	---	---
Vitamin A	24.2	11.6	4.8	9.9	38.1	9.7
Vitamin D	6.7	56.7	6.7	---	---	23.3
Vitamin E	5.2	1.7	19.0	43.1	3.4	13.8

DISCUSSION

Among the different available procedures to calculate food intake in a population, a 24-hour diet recall is an optimal and frequently used method in cross-sectional studies for descriptive purposes, as it was in this case [19]. Furthermore, the interviews were carried out by suitably qualified personnel that are able to interpret cooking techniques and dietary patterns, and also evaluate portion sizes, representing an added value that confirms the validity of the results obtained.

The randomly selected sample reflects the epidemiologic characteristics of the average undergraduate student on the campus of the University of Navarre at Pamplona [20, 21]. They are young people aged 18 to 25 who take a wide variety of university studies and mostly live out of their homes, generally sharing an apartment with other students and, to a lesser extent, in residences, owing to their different origins from all over the country. This fact explains, in some way, why the data from the survey is not limited only to the local area, but also to a wider and more comprehensive dimension.

Breakfast should provide 25% of a person's daily calories, and, in addition, is a good opportunity to include food that is essential in a nutritionally balanced diet, such as milk and derivatives (milk, yogurt, cheese, etc.), cereals and derivatives (bread, breakfast cereals, etc.), and fruits and natural juices, together with table sugar, fat, and olive oil, in order to increase its palatability. The inclusion, to a minor extent, of meat and derivatives, eggs, and fish could be considered, since their nutritional relevance as protein is secondary in our dietary pattern, which exceeds the intake of proteins from animal origins [6, 22, 23]. It is important to note that this recommendation should only be applied to calorie intake, as it is unnecessary, and certainly impractical, to try adjusting the rest of the nutrients in the same proportions, since an adequate nutritional status implies having enough nutrient stores to cover possible daily fluctuations in a person's intake [24]. Previously published works on food consumption for breakfast usually refer to what is considered, in our cultural environment, as the first meal (breakfast), and excludes a mid-morning snack. Nevertheless, in order to compare the results, enable firm conclusions, and develop valid strategies for everyone, we should account for the social and cultural connotations in the populations studied; therefore, the "additional breakfast" (mid-morning snack) should also be considered, since it contributes largely as compensation for the first meal regarding nutrient intake [6, 15, 22]. In fact, this chapter notes that, whenever the surveyed students have both meals over the course of a morning (breakfast and mid-morning snack), even when they are qualitatively different, the percentage share corresponding to the morning intake in terms of daily calorie needs was fulfilled. Furthermore, in this case, the quantitative contribution of some minerals (iron, selenium, and phosphorus) and vitamins (thiamine, riboflavin, niacin, vitamin B6, and vitamin C) represents more than half of the daily recommendations.

The analysis of the results highlights that virtually all students have a first meal that basically consists of some combination of dairy products, preferably whole milk (with/without the addition of sugar, coffee, of cocoa powder), together with either cookies/pastry (croissant, sponge cake, etc.), or toast served with butter/jam/olive oil, or breakfast cereals and, to a lesser extent, with fruits or natural juices. The most common type of breakfast, as one out of four undergraduate students reported, consisted exclusively of one glass of whole milk (with the optional addition of sugar, coffee, or cocoa powder) with biscuits or industrial pastries. Subsequently, in a mid-morning break between classes, 54.2% of the students reported the intake of a second meal (mid-morning snack) that basically consisted of a combination of cereals and derivatives, mostly white bread, with cold meat (ham, spicy sausage, etc.), potato omelet (small portion), or cheese and, less frequently, fruits or whole milk with cookies or pastries.

Regarding the unique features of breakfast for the respondents, it is remarkable how milk and dairy products, especially whole milk, represent a staple for breakfast, being the main dietary source of proteins, calcium, iodine, magnesium, zinc, phosphorus, riboflavin, vitamin B12, and vitamin A. Nevertheless, its consumption implies a significant contribution of saturated fat and cholesterol that may be noticeably reduced by the intake of low-fat (or modified fat content) dairy products; sweets, pastries and bakery are the main dietary source of calories, carbohydrates and, largely, SFA and cholesterol; cereals and derivatives (bread, breakfast cereals, etc.) are the main dietary source of fiber, iron, selenium, thiamine, niacin, pyridoxine, folate and vitamin D; fruits and natural juices are the main origin of vitamin C and vitamin E and, to a great extent, fiber. Therefore, the substitution of sweets, pastries and bakery products with cereals and derivatives – food with a high content in complex carbohydrates and calories - and fruits and natural juices – with a high content in bioactive components (pectin, fructose, carotenes, polyphenols, etc.) - would increase the intake of fiber, minerals, and vitamins, as well as functional foods, while reducing the intake of SFA and cholesterol. However, sweets, pastries, and bakery products include quite heterogeneous ingredients, such as flour, milk, eggs, sugar, and fat from different origins (hydrogenated fats, vegetable oils, margarine, etc.) that explain, in large measure, its relatively significant contribution to mineral and vitamin intake [25-28]. Around half of the surveyed respondents reported the addition of sugar or cocoa powder as ingredients to sweeten milk during breakfast, and, to a lower proportion, the ingestion of fat (butter, margarine, etc.) or olive oil, whose palatability flavors certain foods. These dietary components have a high calorie content, although their consumption is usually not excessive; in the case of olive oil, its high content of oleic acid, essential fatty acids (linoleic and linolenic acids), and other minor components (tocopherol, polyphenols, carotenes, etc.) actually make it essential in the diet, so it contributes in a very significant way to the benefits attributed to a Mediterranean diet.

Approximately half of those subjects surveyed reported the consumption, in the time between breakfast and lunch, of a snack with a relatively heterogeneous composition with the purpose of "recovering" from the morning activity. In fact, this snack provided less than 10% of the daily calorie needs; however, it is the "ideal" energy complement for breakfast in order to get the full intake of a quarter of the recommended daily calories. Nearly one in five undergraduate students ate only one piece of fruit over the course of the morning. However, half of those who had mid-morning snacks ate a medium-sized sandwich with cold meat or a small portion of a potato omelet, which implies an extra contribution of cholesterol; this contribution, together with the intake of milk and derivatives and sweets, pastries, and bakery products for breakfast, means that the total cholesterol intake for breakfast/mid-morning snack, mainly in males, is worthy of consideration in relation to the daily reference intake of cholesterol. Therefore, the ingestion of meat and derivatives for the mid-morning snack should be in moderate amounts, or at least account for it in daily diet planning. Additionally, the analysis of these results serves to underscore that the other half of the surveyed students reported not eating any other food after leaving their residences until lunch;

this means that the percent contribution of energy intake over the course of the morning is far from desirable. Obviously, this raises concerns about the potential negative effects on academic performance that these undergraduate students may be experiencing.

Essentially, despite the nutritional relevance of breakfast/mid-morning snacks, undergraduate students show a trend to eat – over the course of the morning – more and more scarce and/or incomplete amounts of food, which are usually of low nutrient quality. Therefore, these young people should be warned and taught that a daily balanced breakfast constitutes a healthy habit for long-term health that should be pursued.

REFERENCES

[1]   López AM, Ortega RM, Quintas ME, Navia B, Requejo AM. Relationship between habitual breakfast and intellectual performance (logical reasoning) in well-nourished schoolchildren of Madrid (Spain). *European Journal of Clinical Nutrition* 2003; 57 (Suppl 1): 49-53.

[2]   Fernández I, Aguilar MV, Mateos CJ, Martinez MC. Breakfast quality and its relationship to the prevalence of overweight and obesity in adolescents in Guadalajara (Spain). *Nutr Hosp* 2011; 26: 952-958.

[3]   Widenhorn-Müller K, Hille K, Klenk J, Weiland U. Influence of having breakfast on cognitive performance and mood in 13- to 20-year-old high school students: results of a crossover trial. *Pediatrics* 2008; 122:279-84.

[4]   Hoyland A, Dye L, Lawton CL. A systematic review of the effect of breakfast on the cognitive performance of children and adolescents. *Nutr Res Rev* 2009; 22:220-43.

[5]   Cooper SB, Bandelow S, Nevill ME. Breakfast consumption and cognitive function in adolescent schoolchildren. *Physiol Behav* 2011; 103:431-9.

[6]   Reeves S, Halsey LG, McMeel Y, Huber JW. Breakfast habits, beliefs and measures of health and wellbeing in a nationally representative UK sample. *Appetite* 2013; 60:51-7.

[7]   Pinto JA, Carvajal A. El desayuno saludable. Nutrición y salud. Instituto de Salud pública. Madrid 2003.

[8]   Nicklas TA, Bao W, Berenson GS. Breakfast consumption affects adequacy of total daily intake. *J Am Diet Assoc* 1993, 93:886-891.

[9]   Ortega RM, Requejo AM, López AM, Andrés P, Quintas ME, Navia B, Izquierdo M, Rivas T. The importance of breakfast in meeting daily

recommended calcium intake in a group of schoolchildren. *J Am Coll Nutr* 1998, 17:19-24.

[10] Nicklas TA, O'Neil CE, Berenson GS. Nutrient contribution of breakfast, secular trends, and the role of ready-to-eat cereals: a review of data from the Bogalusa Heart Study. *Am J Clin Nutr* 1998, (suppl):757-763.

[11] Ishimoto Y, Yoshida M, Nagata K, Yamada H, Hashizume H, Yoshimura N. Consuming breakfast and exercising longer during high school increases bone mineral density in young adult men. *J Bone Miner Metab* 2012; 22. [Epub ahead of print]

[12] Barr SI, DiFrancesco L, Fulgoni VL 3rd. Consumption of breakfast and the type of breakfast consumed are positively associated with nutrient intakes and adequacy of Canadian adults. *J Nutr* 2013; 143:86-92.

[13] Preziosi P, Galán P, Deheeger M, Yacoub N, Drewnowski A. Breakfast type, daily nutrient intakes and vitamin and mineral status of French children, adolescents an adults. *J Am Coll Nutr* 1999, 18:171-178.

[14] Nicklas TA, Reger C, Myers, O'Neil C. Breakfast consumption with and without vitamin-mineral supplement use favourably impacts daily nutrient intake of ninth-grade students. *J Adolesc Health* 2000, 27:314-321.

[15] Farré R, Frasquets I, Martínez MI y Roma R. Dieta habitual de un grupo de adolescentes valencianos. *Nutr Hosp,* 1999, 14:223-230.

[16] Durá T. Breakfast among students of compulsory secondary education. *Nutr Hosp* 2002; 17: 189-196

[17] Centre d'Ensenyament Superior de Nutrició i Dietètica. Programa de cálculo nutricional CESNID 1.0 (Cd-rom). Universitat de Barcelona: McGraw-Hill; 2003.

[18] Food and Nutrition Board, Institute of Medicine, National Academy of Sciences. Dietary References Intakes: Macronutrients, Elements and vitamins (2004). Available at URL: www.nap.edu.

[19] Martínez MA, Alonso A, Egüés N. Sistemas de evaluación del consumo de alimentos. En: Nutrición aplicada y dietoterapia. Muñoz M, Aranceta J, García-Jalón I (eds.) EUNSA. Pamplona. 2004, pp. 67-82.

[20] Durá T, Castroviejo A. Adherence to a Mediterranean diet in a college population. *Nutr Hosp* 2011; 26:602-608.

[21] Durá T. Intake of milk and dairy products in a college population. *Nutr Hosp* 2008; 23:91-96.

[22] Bollat P, Durá T. Dietary model of college students. *Nutr Hosp* 2008; 3:626-7.

[23] De Rufino P, Redondo C, Amigo T, González-Lamuño D, García M. Breakfast and snack of schooled adolescents in Santander. *Nutr Hosp* 2005; 20:217-222.

[24] Cho S, Dietrich M, Brown CJ, Clark CA, Block G. The effect of breakfast type on total daily energy intake and body mass index: results from the Third National Health and Nutrition Examination Survey (NHANES III). *J Am Coll Nutr* 2003; 22:296-302.

[25] Galvin MA, Kiely M, Flynn A. Impact of ready-to-eat breakfast cereal (RTEBC) consumption on adequacy of micronutrient intakes and compliance with dietary recommendations in Irish adults. *Public Health Nutr* 2003; 6:351-63.

[26] Van den Boom A, Serra-Majem L, Ribas L, Ngo J, Pérez-Rodrigo C, Aranceta J, Fletcher R. The contribution of ready-to-eat cereals to daily nutrient intake and breakfast quality in a Mediterranean setting. *J Am Coll Nutr* 2006; 25:135-43.

[27] Peters BS, Verly E Jr, Marchioni DM, Fisberg M, Martini LA. The influence of breakfast and dairy products on dietary calcium and vitamin D intake in postpubertal adolescents and young adults. *J Hum Nutr Diet* 2012; 25:69-74.

[28] Di Giuseppe R, Di Castelnuovo A, Melegari C, De Lucia F, Santimone I, Sciarretta A, Barisciano P, Persichillo M, De Curtis A, Zito F, Krogh V, Donati MB, de Gaetano G, Iacoviello L; Moli-sani Project Investigators. Typical breakfast food consumption and risk factors for cardiovascular disease in a large sample of Italian adults. *Nutr Metab Cardiovasc Dis* 2012; 22:347-54.

In: Focus on Nutrition …
Editor: Teodoro Durá-Travé

ISBN: 978-1-63463-223-2
© 2015 Nova Science Publishers, Inc.

Chapter 9

INTAKE OF MILK AND DAIRY PRODUCTS IN AN UNDERGRADUATE POPULATION

*Teodoro Durá-Travé[1,2], Fidel Gallinas-Victoriano[2],
Ana Amezqueta-Tiraplegui[2],
Arantxa Mosquera-Gorostidi[2]
and Mikel Mendizábal-Díez[2]*

[1]Department of Pediatrics, Faculty of Medicine, University of Navarra,
Pamplona, Spain
[2]Department of Pediatrics, Navarra Hospital Complex,
Pamplona, Spain

ABSTRACT

Objective: To carry out a descriptive study on the consumption of milk and dairy products in an undergraduate population and to analyze their nutritional contribution to the diet of these students.

Material and methods: Registration of food consumption during a school day (24-hour recall) in a random sample of 500 undergraduate students with ages ranging 19-24 years. Gender, age, level of university studies, class timetable, and type of residence were collected from each respondent.

Results: 98.6% of the undergraduate students interviewed referred having consumed some dairy product during the last 24 hours: 92% milk, 60% yogurts, 32.6% cheese, and 13% other products. There were no differences in the frequency of consumption of different dairy products by age, type of residence, level of university studies, or class timetables; low-fat dairy products consumption was higher (p < 0.05) in women. The mean number of dairy products servings was 2.07, being higher among males (p < 0.05) (2.32) as compared to women (1.99). 42.6% had consumed at least 2 servings, with percentage differences (p < 0.05) between both genders. Consumption of low-fat dairy products represented 24.3% of the whole daily consumption of these foods. In the dietary models of undergraduate students, dairy products constitute the main source of calcium and phosphorus, although they provide significant amounts of saturated fat and cholesterol.

Conclusions: Although virtually all undergraduate students consumed milk and dairy products in the course of the day, the mean value of servings consumed would be lower than recommended, particularly among girls. It would be convenient to recommend daily consumption of low fat dairy products (milk and yogurts) and fresh cheese, which would increase minerals and vitamins intake without increasing the calorie and saturated fat and cholesterol intake, as well as avoiding consumption of other dairy products (crème caramel, custard) reach in carbohydrates and cholesterol.

INTRODUCTION

Milk and derivatives (dairy products) are food with high nutritional value, being an important source of proteins of high biological value, minerals and vitamins, although calcium is the main nutrient provided by this food group. The direct relationship between dairy intake and the acquisition of bone mass grants an even more important nutritional value to this group [1-3]. In this way, insufficient dairy intake, especially during the bone mineralization period, could condition the acquisition of an optimal peak bone mass and, consequently, entails a risk factor for osteoporosis and/or osteoporotic fractures in adulthood [4-10].

The daily recommended intake of calcium between 19-50 years of age is 1000 mg/day [11, 12], an amount that is hard to reach in the absence of a sufficient dairy intake (13-15). The *Guía de la Alimentación Saludable* (Guide for healthy feeding), developed by the Sociedad Española de Nutrición Comunitaria (Spahish Society of Community Nutrition) recommends a daily intake of 2-3 dairy servings or equivalent with an estimated ingestion of 250-300 mg of calcium, except for concrete physiological situations (pregnancy and breastfeeding, athletics, etc.). Nevertheless, the bioavailability of calcium and, consequently, its benefit in the bone is not equivalent among the different dairy products; the utilization of calcium is higher in those products with an increased calcium/proteins and calcium/phosphorus ratio [1, 15].

The individual food consumption surveys reveal that milk and derivatives intake in the Spanish population is characterized by a maximum amount in childhood that progressively decreases in adolescence and later stages in life [16, 17]; this is a fact that can limit the maximum content in bone mineral that is presumably reached at age 24-25. This nutritional impairment justifies the interest to assess milk and derivatives consumption in those segments of the population whose bone mineralization process is still in a critical situation [7, 18], as it occurs in undergraduate population.

The purpose of this chapter is to undertake a descriptive study on milk and derivatives consumption in a undergraduate population and to analyze its nutritional contribution in the diet of these students.

MATERIAL AND METHODS

A nutritional survey was conducted in a randomly selected sample of 500 undergraduate students from the different schools and Faculties in the campus of the University of Navarre at Pamplona (Architecture, Sciences, Law, Human Dietetics and Nutrition, Nursery, Economics, Pharmacy, Literature, Medicine and Journalism) in the course of the second semester of the 2005/2006 academic year. Surveys were carried out by means of personal interviews with students of the final grade of the degree in Human Dietetics and Nutrition of the cited University. The method they applied was the registration of food intake in a school day or "24 hour recall". The interviewer asked in detail about the dairy intake in every meal of the previous day (breakfast, mid-morning snack, lunch, afternoon snack and dinner). In addition, other data from the respondent were registered: sex, age, university studies, class schedule (morning, afternoon or both) and type of residence (student apartment, family home of student residence).

The following amounts of dairy products were defined as standard servings: milk (200 ml), yogurt (250 g), curd-junket (150 g), semi cured cheese (60 g), fresh cheese (120 g), smoothies (250 ml) and ice cream (200 ml). The evaluation of the size of the corresponding servings of dairy products referred by the respondents required the use of a photograph album [19].

The intake of calorie, as well as proteins, carbohydrates, fat, PUFA, MUFA, SFA, cholesterol, calcium and phosphorus was evaluated by calculating the addition of the amount of products divided by the frequency of consumption and the standard amount in every serving of the registered food and its composition in nutrients for every 100 g of edible portion (Programa de Cálculo Nutricional, CESNID 1.0 software) [20]. The calculation of the nutrients that correspond to the different varieties of cheese was individually done, however it has been gathered in the generic term "cheese" for practical reasons.

Results are displayed as means and percentages, with corresponding confidence intervals (95% CI). The statistical analysis (comparison of proportions, Student's t and Chi-square) was done by means of the SPSS 14.0 for Windows software.

RESULTS

The age of the undergraduate students ranged from 19 to 24 years, being 21.1 the average age (95% CI: 21.0-21.2). The distribution by age was: 19 years (n=46), 20 years (n=81), 21 years (n=238), 22 years (n=42), 23 years (n=83) and 24 years (n=10). Table 1 sets forth the distribution of undergraduate students according to sex, type of residence and schedule. Females (76%) prevail over males (24%), but there are no significant differences between type of residence and schedule among sexes.

Table 1. Distribution of undergraduate students according to sex, type of residence and Schedule

	Males n (%)	Females n (%)	Total n (%)
TYPE OF RESIDENCES			
Student apartment	65 (54.2)	211 (55.5)	276 (55.2)
Family home	42 (35.0)	114 (30.0)	156 (31.2)
Student residence	13 (10.8)	55 (14.5)	68 (13.6)
SCHEDULE			
Morning	35 (29.2)	89 (23.4)	124 (24.8)
Afternoon	26 (21.7)	68 (17.9)	94 (18.8)
Both	59 (49.1)	223 (58.6)	282 (56.4)

The results show that 98.6% of the undergraduate students surveyed reported the ingestion of any dairy product in the previous 24 hours. Table 2 illustrates and compares the consumption frequencies of the different milk products among sexes. Overall, 92% of the students referred milk intake, mainly whole milk, and, to a lesser extent, skim or semi skim milk. The frequency of skim milk intake was significantly higher (p<0.05) in females. In addition, 60% took yogurts, mainly plain yogurt, but also fruit or fat free yogurts. The frequency of consumption of plain yogurts was significantly higher (p<0.05) in males, whereas the frequency of consumption of fat free yogurts was significantly higher (p<0.05) in females. The intake of cheese was reported by 32.6% of them, with no differences between sexes. Furthermore, 13% had taken other dairy products, being its frequency significantly higher (p<0.05) in males, mainly as junket and custard. There were no statistically significant differences in the frequency of consumption of the different milk products with regard to age, type of residence, university studies or schedule.

Table 2. Consumption frequencies (%) for the different milk products

MILK PRODUCT	Males	Females	Total
TOTAL MILK	85.8	93.9	92.0
Whole milk	72.5	68.4	69.4
Semi skimmed milk	12.5	11.6	11.8
Skimmed milk*	1.7	17.4	13.6
TOTAL YOGURT	65.9	58.2	60.0
Plain yogurt*	48.3	34.5	39.8
Fruit yogurt	19.2	14.7	15.8
Fat free yogurt*	1.7	9.2	7.4
CHEESE	30.0	33.4	32.6
OTHER PRODUCT *	22.5	10.0	13.0
Junket*	5.8	1.3	2.4
Smoothies	2.5	6.1	5.2
Custard*	15.0	4.7	7.2
Ice cream	2.5	3.9	3.6

(*) (p<0.05)

Figure 1 exposes the distribution of the consumption of the different milk products in the course of the day. As for breakfast, 86% of the students surveyed reported the ingestion of milk and, to a lesser degree, yogurt (3.8%), cheese (2.4%) and other milk products (0.2%). In mid-morning snack, 10.6% have had milk, and, in a lesser proportion, cheese (3%), yogurt (2.6%) and other products (0.4%). In lunch, 25.8% have taken yogurts, other milk products (5.8%), cheese (4.2%) and milk (3.6%). In afternoon snack, 11.6% reported milk, yogurt (4.4%), cheese (3.6%) and other products (2%). As for dinner, the students referred yogurt (32.6%), cheese (18.4%), other products

(5%) and milk (5.8%). In sum, 96.4% of the students reported the intake of milk products in breakfast and, in a smaller proportion, in dinner (61.5%), lunch (39.4%), afternoon snack (21.6%) and mid-morning snack (16.6%).

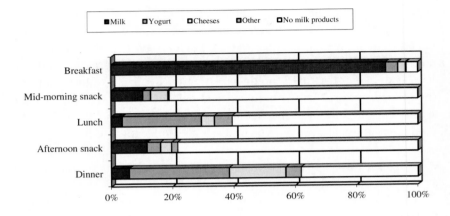

Figure 1. Distribution of the consumption of the different milk products in the course of the day.

Table 3. Average amount of ingestion (milk products) distributed by sex

MILK PRODUCT	Males	Females	Total
TOTAL MILK (ml)*	265.1	242.8	248.8
Whole milk*	233.4	174.8	188.8
Semi skimmed milk	28.3	29.7	29.4
Skimmed milk*	3.3	38.9	30.6
YOGURT (g)*	110.4	86.5	92.2
Plain yogurt*	76.1	51.6	57.5
Fruit yogurt	32.3	21.1	23.8
Fat free yogurt*	2.1	13.8	11.0
CHEESE	18.9	16.2	16.9
OTHER PRODUCT (g)	8.3	1.9	3.4
Junket*	2.5	10.8	8.8
Smoothies*	28.6	9.8	14.3
Custard*	3.7	6.4	5.8
Ice cream			
	438.8	372.6	388.5
TOTAL AMOUNT (g)*			

(*) (p<0.05)

Table 3 shows and compares the average values for the intake of the different milk products registered between sexes. Males had taken total amounts of milk and yogurt significantly higher (p<0.05), as well as junket and custard; meanwhile, females have had higher amounts of fat free milk products (milk and yogurts) and smoothies. The total quantity of dairy product intake was significantly higher (p<0.05) in males.

Table 4. Average values for the number of milk product servings according to sex, type of residence and schedule

SEX		
Males	Females	Total
2.32 (1.21)*	1.99 (0.8)*	2.07 (0.93)
TYPE OF RESIDENCE		
Family home	Student apartment	Student residence
2.19 (1.03)	2.00 (0.93)	2.02 (0.86)
SCHEDULE		
Morning	Afternoon	Both
2.06 (0.97)	2.15 (0.85)	2.06 (0.93)

(*) (p<0.05)

Table 4 outlines and compares the average value for the number of milk product servings consumed. The number of milk product servings was significantly higher (p<0.05) in males, showing no significant differences in relation to the type of residence or schedule. Furthermore, 42.6% of surveyed students reported less than 2 servings (males: 36.7%, females: 44.5%), 38% 2 servings (males: 30.8%, females: 40.3%), 13.8% 3 servings (males: 19.2%, females: 12.1%) and, finally, 5.6% 4 or more servings (males: 13.3%, males: 3.2%), showing significant differences (p<0.05) between sexes.

From the total amount of milk products consumed, milk (whole: 48.6%, semi skimmed milk: 7.6% and fat free: 7.8%) together with yogurt (whole milk: 21% and fat free: 2.8%) represented 87.7%, whereas other milk products (8.4%) and cheese (4.4%) accounted for a lower proportion. There were no significant differences between sexes, except for fat free milk, whose percentage contribution was significantly higher in females (females: 10.4%, males: 0.8%).

Table 5 displays and compares the mean values for the intake of calories, immediate principles, cholesterol, calcium and phosphorus corresponding to the milk products between sexes. This intake was significantly higher (p<0.05) in males. In the same way, the percentage values of calories and nutrients provided by milk products in relation to the reference values (%DRIs). The fatty acids provided by milk products were mainly SFA (62%) and, in a smaller proportion, MUFA (29.3%) and PUFA (8.7%), with no percentage differences among sexes.

Table 5. Average value of the calorie and nutrient intake provided by milk products in both sexes, and percentage provided in relation to references (%DRI)

NUTRIENTS	Males X (IC 95%)	%DRI	Females X (IC 95%)	%DRI
Energy (kcal)	380.9 (16.2)*	12.7	306.7 (9.3)*	13.3
Proteins (g)	20.9 (2.1)*	37.3	17.9 (1.1)*	38.9
Carbohydrates (g)	29.4 (2.7)*	22.6	23.2 (1.1)*	17.8
Fat (g)	20.7 (2.3)*	---	16.3 (1.8)*	---
Cholesterol (mg)	95.0 (6.6)*	31.7	62.6 (3.0)*	20.9
Calcium (mg)	637.1 (39.0)*	63.7	560.2 (19.2)*	56.0
Phosphorus (mg)	505.3 (24.0)*	72.2	438,8 (11.7)*	62.7

(*) (p<0.05)

Table 6. Percentage contribution (%) to the nutrient intake for every milk product consumed

	MILK	YOGURT	CHEESE	OTHER
Calorie	45.8	19.2	23.7	11.3
Proteins	48.8	15.5	29.5	6.3
Carbohydrate	51.6	26.0	0.4	22.0
Fat	59.4	10.0	25.5	5.0
SFA	50.5	13.8	29.4	6.4
MUFA	50.0	13.0	30.4	6.5
PUFA	14.3	4.3	78.6	3.6
Cholesterol	44.0	12.2	19.2	24.6
Calcium	51.2	19.2	23.9	5.7
Phosphorus	53.0	20.7	18.4	7.9

Table 6 displays the percentage contribution of the consumption of the different milk products in the calorie and nutrient intake. Milk provided proportionally the biggest amount of nutrients, except for PUFA (14.3%). Yogurt provided a considerable proportion of carbohydrates (26%) and phosphorus (20.7%). Cheese contributed with proteins (29.5%), fat (25.5%), especially as PUFA, calories (23.7%) and calcium (23.9%). The remaining dairy products contributed mainly with cholesterol (24.6%) and carbohydrates (22%).

DISCUSSION

Among the different methods available to assess food consumption in a concrete population, the 24-hour recall surveys are an optimal and widely used method in cross-sectional studies with descriptive purposes, as in this case [21]. Furthermore, the completion of surveys by qualified interviewers, able to interpret cooking techniques, consumption patterns and serving sizes, represents an additional value that proves the validity of the results obtained. Nevertheless, a photograph album of servings and food portions was also used to dispel the reasonable doubts that may arise in relation to the amount of food ingested.

The random sample reflects the epidemiological characteristics of the standard undergraduate student in the campus of the University of Navarre at Pamplona. The average student is 19 to 24 years old, takes a wide variety of university degrees and, in a large proportion, lives in an apartment with other fellow students and has a schedule that includes morning and afternoon.

The analysis of food consumption of the different milk products that have been registered outlines how the majority of the undergraduate students take milk products in the course of the day, being whole milk a food staple in breakfast and yogurt −also made with whole milk- a quite common food in lunch and/or dinner. Meanwhile, the ingestion of other milk products, including the different types of cheese, was comparatively minor. Additionally, with the exception of sex, no other variable (age, type of residence, schedule and grade) has a significant influence on food preferences in the group of milk products.

Even when the average consumption of milk and dairy products in the studied population substantially surpasses the references from other authors [22-27], 42.6% of these students consumed less than two daily portions of milk products. In general terms, the consumption of milk products among undergraduate students, regardless of the type of residence and schedule, would be limited to a glass of whole milk for breakfast and a full-fat yogurt for lunch or dinner. These results match the data provided by different studies on milk products consumption in Spanish population and, consequently, confirm that a significant percentage of undergraduate students consume an amount of product from this food group below the references for this age group and, especially within females [16, 17, 28, 29]. It is to be noted that a continued consumption of milk products below the recommendations makes the addition of calcium/dietary supplements necessary [1, 2, 8, 30], since this situation does not guarantee a normal rate of bone mineralization.

Milk and derivatives are food with a high nutritional value, and the peculiarity that some of the nutritional components have an additional functional activity with beneficial effects for the consumer health [31, 32], even when this food group might imply a significant intake of saturated fat and cholesterol. Although the consumption of dairy products might seem adequate given its high percent contribution in calcium and phosphorus with respect to the established recommendations, the diversity of milk products consumed by undergraduate students has a series of peculiarities which should be noted. On one hand, milk products are the main dietary source of calcium and phosphorus, as well as an important source of proteins that, to a large extent, have prompted us to consider their daily consumption as mandatory [33-35]. However, this dietary model that has been adopted by undergraduate student implies a considerable intake of fat, mainly as SFA, and cholesterol, which could be significantly reduced by the consumption of low fat or modified fatty composition products. On the other hand, it is pertinent to note how the intake of other milk products, such as custard or pudding/crème caramel, despite the comparatively low percent contribution to the total amount of dairy products consumed by undergraduate students, represents a significant percent contribution of carbohydrates and cholesterol that should obviously be restricted.

The consumption of fat free milk products among undergraduate students barely represents 24.3% of the total daily amount of milk products intake. In this sense, it is a requirement to suggest the intake of fat free/low fat milk products (milk and yogurt) to these group of the population, as well as the consumption of the different varieties of fresh cheese available in the market (Burgos style, petit Suisse, mozzarella, cottage-ricotta style cheese, etc.). This intervention would increase the intake of minerals and vitamins without increasing the intake of calories and/or SFA and cholesterol. In addition, the consumption of other milk products (custard, crème caramel), which have a high content in carbohydrates and cholesterol should be avoided [36-38].

As a conclusion, the consumption – both qualitative and quantitative – of milk and derivatives in the undergraduate population is inadequate; consequently, it should be considered to spread clear information on the nutritional importance of this food group among undergraduate students, as well as the knowledge of dietary alternatives available in the market, such as low fat milk products with a high density in mineral and vitamins, which could contribute substantially to the intake of dietary calcium required for the acquisition of an adequate peak bone mass, as well as other nutrients with beneficial effects on consumer health.

REFERENCES

[1]   Weinsier RL, Krumdieck CL. Dairy foods and bone health: examination evidence. *Am J Clin Nutr* 2000; 72:68-1-689.

[2]   Merrilees MJ, Smart EJ, Gilchrist NL, et al. Effects of diary food supplements on bone mineral density in teenage girls. *Eur J Nutr* 2000; 39:256-62.

[3]   Huth PJ, DiRienzo DB, Miller GD. Major scientific advances with dairy foods in nutrition and health. *J Dairy Sci* 2006; 89:1207-21.

[4]   Bachrach LK. Bone mineralization in childhood and adolescents. *Curr Opin Pediatr* 1993; 5:467-473.

[5]   Del Rio L, Carrascosa M, Pons F, Gussinye M, Yeste D, Domenech FM. Bone mineral density of the lumbar spine in Caucasian Mediterranean Spanish children and adolescents. Changes related to age, sex and puberty. *Pediatr Res* 1994; 35: 362-366.

[6]   Boot AM, Rider MAJ, Pols HA, Krenning EP, Muinck PF. Bone mineral density in children and adolescents: relation to puberty, calcium intake and physical activity. *J Clin Endocrinol Metab* 1997; 82:57-62.

[7]   Borrajo E, Gutierrez A, Gutierrez E. Ostoporosis. En: *Metabolismo fosfocálcico*. Dieguez C, Iturriaga R, eds. McGraw-Hill-Interamericana. Madrid. 2003. pp. 113-131.

[8]   Murray TM. Prevention and management of osteoporosis: consensus statements from the Scientific Advisory Board of the Osteoporosis Society of Canada. Calcium nutrition and osteoporosis. *CMAJ* 1996; 155:935-9.

[9]   Infante D, Tormo R. Risk of inadequate bone mineralization in diseases involving long-term suppression of dairy products. *J Pediatr Gastroenterol Nutr* 2000; 30:310-313.

[10]   Lutz J, Tesar R. Mother-daugther pairs: spinal and femoral bone densities and dietary intake. *Am J Clin Nutr* 1999; 52:872-877.

[11]   Greer FR, Krebs NF. Optimizing bone health and calcium intakes of infants, children, and adolescents. *Pediatrics* 2006; 117:578-85.

[12]   Dietary Reference Intakes for Energy, Carbohydrate, Fiber, Fat, Fatty Acids, Cholesterol, Protein and Amino Acids. Food and Nutrition Board, Institute of Medicine, National Academies (2002). www.nap.edu

[13]   Lanou AJ, Berkow SE, Barnard ND. Calcium, dairy products, and bone health in children and young adults: a reevaluation of the evidence. *Pediatrics* 2005; 115:736-43.

[14]   Ballabriga A, Carrascosa A. M*asa ósea y nutrición*. En: Ballabriga A, Carrascosa A. Nutrición en la Infancia y Adolescencia. Madrid. E. Ergón, S.A. 1998. pp. 431-452.

[15]   Ortega RM, MENA MC, López AM. *Leche y lácteos: valor nutricional*. En: Leche, lácteos y salud. Aranceta J, Serra L, eds. Ed. Médica-Panamericana. Madrid. 2005. pp. 19-30.

[16]   Aranceta J. *La leche y los lácteos en la alimentación de los españoles*. En: Leche, lácteos y salud. Aranceta J, Serra L, eds. Ed. Médica-Panamericana. Madrid. 2005. pp. 31-41.

[17]   Serra L, Aranceta J. *Alimentación infantil y juvenil*. Estudio enkid. Vol. 3. Ed. Masson S.A. Barcelona. 2002. pp. 1-195.

[18]   Nicklas TA. Calcium intake trends and health consequences from childhood through adulthood. *J Am Coll Nutr* 2003; 22:340-56.

[19]   Portions Alimentaires. *Manuel photos pour l'estimation des quantites*. Ed. Politécnica. Paris. 1994.

[20]   Farran A, Zamora R, Cervera P. *Tablas de Composición de Alimentos del CESNID*. Ed. McGraw-Hill-Interamericana. Madrid. 2003.

[21]   Martinez MA, Alonso A, Egüés N. *Sistemas de evaluación del consumo de alimentos*. En: Nutrición aplicada y dietoterapia. Muñoz M, Aranceta J, García-Jalón I, eds. EUNSA. Pamplona. 2004. pp. 67-82.

[22]   Muñoz KA, Krebs-Smith SM, Ballard-Barbash R, Cleveland LE. Foods intakes of US children and adolescents compared with recommendations. *Pediatrics* 1997; 100:323-329.

[23]   Klesges RC, Harmon-Clayton K, Ward KD, et al. Predictors of milk consumption in a population of 17- to 35-year-old military personnel. *J Am Diet Assoc* 1999; 99:821-6.

[24] Gonzalez CA, Argilaga S, Agudo A, et al. Sociodemographic differences in adherence to the Mediterranean dietary pattern in Spanish populations. *Gac Sanit* 2002; 16: 214-21.

[25] Auld G, Boushey CJ, Bock MA, et al. Perspectives on intake of calcium-rich foods among Asian, Hispanic, and white preadolescent and adolescent females. *J Nutr Educ Behav* 2002; 34:242-51.

[26] Wham CA, Worsley A. New Zealanders' attitudes t milk: implications for public health. *Public Health Nutr* 2003; 6:73-8.

[27] Novotny R, Boushey C, Bock MA, et al. Calcium intake of Asian, Hispanic and white youth. *J Am Coll Nutr* 2003; 22:64-70.

[28] Fulgoni VL 3rd, Huth PJ, DiRienzo DB, Miller GD. Determination of the optimal number of dairy servings to ensure a low prevalence of inadequate calcium intake in Americans. *J Am Coll Nutr* 2004; 23: 651-9.

[29] Matkovic V, Kostial K, Simonovic I, Buzin R, Brodarec A. Factors that influence peak bone mass in adolescents females. *Am J Clin Nutr* 1999; 52:878-888.

[30] Heaney R, Dowell M, Rafferty K, Bierman J. Bioavailability of the calcium in fortified soy imitation milk, with some observations on method. *Am J Clin Nutr* 2000; 71:1166-1169.

[31] Baró L, López-Huertas E, Boza JJ. Leche y derivados lácteos. En: Tratado de Nutrición. Angel Gil-Hernández, ed. *Ed. Grupo Acción Médica.* Madrid. 2005. pp. 79-105.

[32] Huth PJ, DiRienzo DB, Miller GD. Major scientific advances with dairy foods in nutrition and health. *J Dairy Sci.* 2006; 89:1207-1221.

[33] Helsing E. Traditional diets and disease patterns of the Mediterranean, circa 1960. *Am J Clin Nutr* 1995; 61 (Suppl):1329-1337.

[34] Ferro-Luzzi A, Branca F. Mediterranean diet, Italian-style: prototype of a healthy diet. *Am J Clin Nutr* 1995; 61(Suppl): 1338-1345.

[35] Willet WC, Sacks F, Trichopoulou A et al. Mediterranean diet pyramid: a cultural model for healthy eating. *Am J Clin Nutr* 1995; 61(Suppl): 1402-1406.

[36] Aranceta J, Serra L, Pérez C, Mataix J. *Leche y lácteos: guía para el consumo.* En: Leche, lácteos y salud. Aranceta J, Serra Ll, eds. Editorial Médica Panamericana, S.A. Madrid. 2005. pp. 143-148.

[37] Weinberg LG, Berner LA, Groves JE. Nutrient contributions of dairy foods in the United States, Continuing Survey of Food Intakes by Individuals, 1994-1996, 1998. *J Am Diet Assoc* 2004; 104:895-902.

[38] Ranganathan R, Nicklas TA, Yang SJ, Berenson GS. The nutritional impact of dairy product consumption on dietary intakes of adults (1995-1996): the Bogalusa Heart Study. *J Am Diet Assoc.* 2005; 105:1391-1400.

In: Focus on Nutrition …
Editor: Teodoro Durá-Travé

ISBN: 978-1-63463-223-2
© 2015 Nova Science Publishers, Inc.

Chapter 10

QUALITY OF DIETARY HABITS (ADHERENCE TO MEDITERRANEAN DIET) IN AN UNDERGRADUATE POPULATION

Teodoro Durá-Travé[1,2], Fidel Gallinas-Victoriano[2], Monserrat Elso-Fábregas[2], Noelia Ulibarrena-Ascarza[2] and Ibone Vaquero-Iñigo[2]

[1]Department of Pediatrics, Faculty of Medicine, University of Navarra, Pamplona, Spain
[2]Department of Pediatrics, Navarra Hospital Complex, Pamplona, Spain

ABSTRACT

Objective: To determine the adherence to Mediterranean diet of an undergraduate population and to analyze several factors that could condition its nutritional quality.

Material and methods: Distribution of the Kidmed test to a random sample of 570 undergraduate students. The Kidmed index (0-12) showed whether the adherence to Mediterranean diet was low (0-3), intermediate (4-7) or high (8-12). Sex, age, weight, height, and body mass index were gathered from each participant, as well as the type of residence and the province of origin.

Results: The sample consisted in 217 males and 353 females aged 18-25 years. Overall, 9.5% of the undergraduate students had a low

Kidmed index, 62.1% intermediate, and 28.4% high. Those students living at their family home had a high percentage of adherence (35.6%), significantly higher (p < 0.05) than those living at a student residence (11.1%) or at a student apartment (11.2%). Overweight students had a low percentage of adherence (15.5%), significantly higher (p < 0.05) than those with a normal nutritional status (8.5%).

Conclusions: The results show that 71.6% of undergraduate students need to improve their dietary pattern (low to intermediate adherence to Mediterranean diet), and we observe a certain family factor of preservation of the traditional dietary habits. Those undergraduate students with low adherence present a higher risk for being overweight. It would be convenient to develop nutritional education programs in the university curricula.

INTRODUCTION

Traditional diet from Mediterranean area countries is characterized by a frequent consumption of vegetables, legumes, fruits, dried fruits and nuts, food grain and, specially highlighted, olive oil. In addition to this, there is a moderate consumption of fish, eggs and dairy products, mainly yogurt and cheese, and a minor consumption of meat and animal fat [1-4]. Mediterranean diet not only guarantees an adequate caloric and nutritional intake but it also contributes to prevent cardiovascular and degenerative diseases, diabetes, cancer and others and, on the whole, to a higher life expectancy [5-11].

The modernization of society implies a series of sociological and/or cultural changes which unavoidably affect food habits and preferences. People devote less time to food shopping and elaboration and, instead, processed food is preferred over home made food. In general, this entails an excessive consumption of animal products, mainly meat and derivatives, and refined sugar, consequently increasing the amount of saturated fat and cholesterol in the diet [12-17].

This virtual damage of dietary patterns has begun a fear about the slow disappearance of the Mediterranean diet [13, 18, 19]. This would justify, in large measure, the study of the quality of dietary habits in general population with a special focus on those sectors that can be influenced more easily like, as an example, the youth. In order to evaluate the degree of adherence to Mediterranean diet, several *evaluation indexes* have been developed based on qualitative and/or quantitative aspects. Those aspects were related to the consumption of the different "typical" components of the Mediterranean diet which generally require a laborious process of information gathering on food consumption [6, 8, 13, 20-24]. At present day, the test for Mediterranean diet quality assessment or Kidmed index [25] is available to quickly determine the degree of adherence to Mediterranean diet and its usefulness has been successfully matched [26-30].

The objective of the present chapter consists in determining the adherence to Mediterranean diet of an undergraduate population and analyzing diverse factors which could condition its nutritional quality.

MATERIAL AND METHODS

Adherence to Mediterranean diet patterns has been evaluated by applying *Kidmed Mediterranean diet adherence test* [25] to a random sample of 570 undergraduate students from different faculties of the campus of the University of Navarre at Pamplona (Science, Nursing, Pharmacy and Medicine) during the second semester of the 2008/2009 academic year. The distribution of questionnaires or kidmed test was personally performed by final year students of the Degree in Human Nutrition and Dietetics from the University itself. Sex, age, anthropometric variables (weight, height and BMI), type of residence (student apartment, family home or student residence) and province of origin were also recorded from every survey respondent. According to their province origin, the respondents were divided into the following geographical areas: Navarra, North (Galicia, Asturias, Cantabria and the Basque Country), Northeast (Aragon, Catalonia and Balearic Islands), Centro (Castilla-León, Madrid, Castilla-La Mancha, La Rioja and Extremadura) and East (Valencia, Murcia, Andalusia and the Canary Islands). Those from foreign origins were excluded (the questionnaire was not distributed).

The body mass index (BMI) was calculated using the formula: weight (kg) / height^2 (m). According to the BMI value, four groups were defined: (1) Undernourishment, when the score was less than 18.5. (2) Normality, if it ranged between 18.5 and 24.99. (3) Overweight, if it ranged between 25 and 29.99. (4) Obesity, if it was above 30.

The kidmed test [25] consists of 16 questions which must be answered in the affirmative / negative way (yes / no). Affirmative answers to the questions that represent a positive aspect in relation to Mediterranean diet (they are 12) add 1 point, and affirmative answers on the questions representing a negative connotation in relation to Mediterranean diet (there are 4) subtract 1 point. The total score results in kidmed index, which is classified into three categories:

a)   8-12: Optimum Mediterranean (high adherence).
b)   4 to 7: Need to improve the dietary patterns to suit the Mediterranean
      model (medium adherence).
c)   0 to 3: Low quality diet (low adherence).

Results are shown as means and percentages with confidence intervals
(95% CI). Statistical analysis (comparison of proportions, Student t and Chi-
square) was performed using the SPSS 17.0 for Windows (Chicago, USA)
software.

Table 1. Distribution of undergraduate students by sex, type of residence, geographical origin and nutritional status

	Males n (%)	Females n (%)	Total n (%)
Type of residence			
Student apartment	107 (49.3)	171 (48.4)	278 (48.8)
Family home	59 (27.2)	116 (32.9)	175 (30.7)
Student residence	51 (23.5)	66 (18.7)	117 (20.5)
Geographical origin			
Navarra	75 (35.9)	141 (40.9)	216 (39.0)
North	49 (23.4)	96 (27.8)	145 (26.2)
North East	32 (15.3)	35 (10.1)	67 (12.1)
Centre	33 (15.8)	43 (12.5)	76 (13.7)
South East	20 (9.6)	30 (8.5)	50 (9.0)
Nutritional status*			
Undernourishment	6 (2.8)	25 (7.4)	42 (7.6)
Normal	167 (78.8)	281 (83.1)	437 (79.5)
Overweight	37 (17.5)	31 (9.2)	68 (12.9)
Obesity	2 (0.9)	1(0.3)	3 (0.5)

(*) p<0.05

RESULTS

The sample obtained was composed of 353 females (61.9%) and 217 males (38.1%). The age of the undergraduate survey respondents ranged between 18 and 25 years, with an average age of 20.6 years (95% CI: 20.4-20.8). The age distribution was: 18-19 years (n = 200), 20-21 years (n = 185), 22-23 years (n = 152) and 24-25 years (n = 33). Table 1 shows the distribution by sex, type of residence, geographical origin and nutritional status. There were no significant percentage differences between type of residence and geographical origin among both sexes. However, some males showed overweight / obesity (18.4%) percentages significantly higher (p <0.05) than those in females (9.5%). BMI of males was 23.3 (95% CI: 23.0-23.6) being significantly higher (p <0.05) than that in females which was 21.0 (95% CI: 20.8-21.2).

Kidmed test results of both sexes are presented and compared in Table 2. Of the total sample, 9.5% of respondents had a low Kidmed index score, 62.1% an intermediate index score and 28.4% a higher index score; being the average value of the Kidmed index 6.17 (95% CI :6.02-6.32). Although there were no significant differences between the mean values of the Kidmed index between sexes (females 6.3 and males 6.0), the percentage of men with low adherence to Mediterranean diet was significantly higher (12.9%) than that in women (7.4%).There were also statistically significant differences (p <0.05) between sexes in several items. Males attend burger restaurants (fast food) at least once a week, eat legumes more than once a week, have pasta or rice almost daily, take nuts at least 2 or 3 times a week, eat bakery for breakfast and take two yogurts and / or cheese every day (more often than females); females have fresh or cooked vegetables at least once a day and have cereals or derivatives (bread, toast, etc..) for breakfast (more often than males).

Table 3 presents and compares the degree of adherence to Mediterranean diet (Kidmed index) in relation to the type of residence and nutritional status of the undergraduate respondents. Those living in a family home had high percentages of adherence to the Mediterranean diet (35.6%). They were significantly higher (p <0.05) than those who lived in a student residence (25%) or a student apartment (23%); in contrast, those who lived in a residence (11.1%) or student apartment (11.2%) show lower percentage values of adherence to Mediterranean diet in higher rates (p <0.05) than those who lived in family residence (5.7%). Undergraduate students living in their family home had an average value of kidmed test of 6.6 (95% CI: 6.3-6. 9) that was significantly higher (p <0.05) than those living in a student residence: 6.1

(95% CI: 5.7-6. 5) or a student apartment: 5.9 (95% CI: 5.6-6. 2). The BMI of the undergraduates living in their family home was 21.4 (95% CI: 21.0-21. 8), which is significantly lower than that of the students living in a residence: 22.3 (95% CI: 22.0-22. 6) or a student apartment: 22.5 (95% CI: 22.2-22. 8). Overweight students had low percentage values of adherence to Mediterranean diet (15.5%) in significantly higher (p <0.05) rates than those students whose nutritional status was normal (8.5%).

No statistically significant differences in the kidmed index related to age, university studies and geographical origin (excluding Navarra due to its highest proportion of undergraduates living in their family home) were observed.

Table 2. Test on quality of Mediterranean diet according to sex

Test Kidmed	Males (%)	Females (%)	Total (%)
Takes a fruit or fruit juice everyday	72.4	75.9	74.6
Has a second fruit or fruit juice everyday	31.3	32.6	32.1
Has fresh or cooked vegetables regularly once per day*	52.1	68.3	62.1
Has fresh or cooked vegetables more than once a day*	12.0	21.8	18.1
Consumes fish regularly (at least 2 or 3 times a week)	49.8	56.9	54.2
Goes more than once a week to a fast-food (hamburger) restaurant *	33.2	13.9	21.2
Likes pulses and eats them more than once a week*	78.3	64.0	69.5
Consumes pasta or rice almost every day (5 or more times per week)*	47.0	22.7	31.9
Has cereals or grains (bread, etc) for breakfast*	78.8	86.7	83.1
Consumes nuts regularly (at least 2- 3 times per week)*	33.2	24.1	27.5
Uses olive oil at home	72.5	73.8	73.2
Skips breakfast	19.8	15.0	16.8
Has a dairy product for breakfast (milk, yogurt, etc)	92.2	91.8	91.9
Has commercially baked goods or pastries for breakfast*	23.6	12.2	16.5
Takes 2 yogurt and/or some cheese (40 g) daily*	53.9	43.9	47.7
Takes sweets and candy several times every day	16.1	15.0	15.4
Kidmed index*			
≤3 (low adherence)	12.9	7.4	9.5
4-7 (intermediate adherence)	60.8	62.9	62.1
≥8 (high adherence)	26.3	29.7	28.4

(*) p<0.05.

Table 3. Degree of adherence to Mediterranean diet (Kidmed index) in relation to the type of residence and nutritional status.

Kidmed index	Low %	Medium %	High %
Type of residence			
Family home	5.7	58.7	35.6
Student residence	11.1	63.9	25.0
Student apartment	11.2	65.8	23.0
Nutritional status*			
Undernourishment	9.5	64.3	26.2
Normal	8.5	62.4	29.1
Overweight	15.5	57.7	26.8

(*) $p < 0.05$

DISCUSSION

The *evaluation indexes* for the assessment of the quality of Mediterranean diet came from the need of having tools that allow evaluating and, more specifically, determining the degree of adherence to Mediterranean dietary patterns of the population [6, 8, 13, 20-23, 31]; in fact, several indexes have been developed and used attending qualitative and / or quantitative facts of the consumption of various "typical" components of the Mediterranean diet [24]. Nevertheless, its specificity has been questioned since the term "Mediterranean diet" is somehow imprecise and also its conceptual laxity increases in relation to its known variants [1, 2, 24, 31, 32]; the epidemiological (not experimental) studies have confirmed the importance of the adherence to Mediterranean diet on human health [6, 8, 15, 28, 33] and its relationship with certain life styles [13, 20, 29, 34]. Kidmed test is very easy to fill in by the survey respondent and also very easy to be interpreted by the interviewer. It is drawn from the above indexes and / or principles underpinning the Mediterranean dietary pattern and can quickly determine the degree of adherence to Mediterranean diet in a population [25].The resulting Kidmed index is an instrument that, on one hand, immediately identifies the population with unhealthy eating habits; and, on the other hand, it has been found that a higher score guarantees a supply of nutrients in sufficient amounts and proper proportions, justifying its use [27, 29, 30, 35].

The randomly selected sample reflected the epidemiological characteristics of the average undergraduate student of the University of Navarra [36] at Pamplona. They were young students, between 18 and 25 years old, from different geographical areas of the country, which would explain why a large majority of them were living outside of the family home, usually sharing an apartment with other students and, to a lesser extent, in students residences. This event allows us considering that the data provided are not confined exclusively to this geographical environment but take a broader dimension.

When analyzing the responses to the different items, we notice that only 28.4% of the youth surveyed reported having consistent eating habits that followed the Mediterranean pattern (high adhesion). Being the first time in which the kidmed index has been used in a population of these features -in fact, it has been used almost exclusively in children and adolescents- there are no comparable previous data. The Spanish studies previously published in relation to it show optimal adherence values to the Mediterranean diet being 48.5% [25, 35] for childhood and 42.9% [25, 37] for adolescents, respectively; although these figures are significantly lower in other Mediterranean countries [29, 30]. Given that the undergraduates were teenagers few years earlier, and saving the methodological differences, one might consider the existence of a progressive deterioration of adherence to Mediterranean diet which begins to be noticed in adolescents [37]. In general terms, we note that survey respondents did not reach the recommendations of consumption of most of the foods that are the basis of the Mediterranean diet pyramid, that is to say, fruit (only 32.1% were taking daily a second piece), vegetables (only 18.1% were taking a second helping daily), nuts (just 27.5% were taking them weekly) and pasta or rice (barely 31.9 % were taking them almost daily); furthermore, the consumption of yogurt and / or cheese was also relatively low. On the other hand, it should be emphasized that a relatively large proportion of these young people were having pastry/bakery products for breakfast (16.5% of respondents) or taking sweets daily (15.4% of respondents); and these foods occupy the top of the food pyramid and, therefore, their frequency of consumption should be sporadic. The Mediterranean diet, as well as a prototype of healthy diet, represents a life style circumscribed to a climate and/or geographical area [1-4, 10, 32]. In this sense, the trend of undergraduate students to attend burger restaurants (21.2% of survey respondents would go once or more per week) and / or the lack of regularity at breakfast (16.8% of respondents did not eat breakfast daily) denote largely a loss of cultural heritage represented by the Mediterranean diet. Olive oil is an essential element of Mediterranean culture that inevitably prevails in the different ethnic and / or current Mediterranean countries. To a large extent, olive oil is responsible of the beneficial effects of this dietary pattern [4, 38], which would explain the culinary use of olive oil expressed by respondents in the different types of residence.

Significant differences in the degree of adherence to Mediterranean diet in relation to the type of residence have been observed. While 35.6% of undergraduate students living at their family home had optimal values of kidmed index (high adhesion), barely 23 % of those living in shared apartments with other fellow students (who, by the way, were the majority) reached those values. And while 11.2% of those students living in shared apartments had a very low quality diet (low adhesion), these figures barely reached 5.7% among those who lived with their families. This fact highlights, on one hand, the existence of a certain family conservative factor for the traditional dietary habits and, on the other hand, a trend among undergraduates with more independent lifestyles from their families (due to their different geographical origin) to adopt new patterns of Western dietary habits. These habits are characterized by an increasing consumption of processed food to the detriment of Mediterranean cuisine based on a wide variety of natural and fresh foods. However, although the undergraduate students living with their families enjoyed a greater adherence to Mediterranean diet, a 71.6% of the survey respondents, with no gender differences, showed the need to improve their eating patterns as a result of the loss of some traditional dietary habits. This fact would mean that a significant proportion of undergraduate students have some risk of nutritional lack and/or imbalance [27] and, moreover, raises concerns about a virtual disappearance of the Mediterranean diet in a short and / or medium period [13, 17-19].

Some more significant differences have been noticed in the nutritional status of young people in relation to the degree of adherence to Mediterranean diet. That is, those undergraduate students who showed poorer nutritional quality and / or low adherence to Mediterranean diet had a higher risk of being overweight, which confirms the protective effect on overweight that a balanced diet has (in this particular case, the Mediterranean diet) as it has been pointed out by various authors [8, 28]. And once again, in the case of the undergraduates, the family home would have a positive effect on their nutritional status in contrast to those from other geographical areas living in student residences and especially those living in apartments with other students.

The results underscore the need that the general population has, more specifically undergraduates, of nutritional education. This population group should know that Mediterranean diet, as a prototype of healthy eating pattern, helps maintain optimal health levels and, although it includes all foods, their frequency of use should follow the guidelines in the nutritional pyramid [2]. Therefore, dietary standards for these undergraduate students would basically consist on increasing the daily intake of fresh fruit and vegetables, pasta and / or rice, nuts, dairy products, primarily yogurt and / or cheese and legumes and fish at least 2 or 3 times a week; as well as encouraging the consumption of olive oil as the only cooking fat. On the other hand, we should recommend the occasional consumption of industrial pastries and sweets, and also stress the importance of a daily breakfast that includes cereal, milk and fruits [39].

It should be noted that this study has a number of methodological limitations, since some variables were not recorded. These variables were demographic characteristics, socioeconomic status, level of parental education, physical activity, sedentary habits (nap, television, computers, study time, etc.) and they define the lifestyle of the survey respondents, influencing, to some extent, the degree of adherence to Mediterranean diet [13, 20, 28-30, 40].

It would be convenient to design nutritional education programs in order to get the knowledge for people in general and youth in particular, ready to fit a healthy diet in their lives. In order to do this, governments should promote dietary advice in primary care programs and develop nutritional education programs in formal education. Moreover, and given the transcendental relationship between diet and health, one could envisage the possibility that subjects such as diet and human nutrition could be included in university studies curriculum.

REFERENCES

[1]   Helsing E. Traditional diets and disease patterns of the Mediterranean, circa 1960. *Am J Clin Nutr* 1995; 61(Suppl):1329-37.

[2]   Willet WC, Sacks F, Trichopoulou A, Drescher G, Ferro-Luzzi A, Helsing E, et al. Mediterranean diet pyramid: a cultural model for healthy eating. *Am J Clin Nutr* 1995; 61(Suppl):1402-6.

[3]   Trichopoulou A and Lagiou P. Healthy traditional Mediterranean diet: an expression of culture, history, and lifestyle. *Nutr Rev* 1997; 55:383-9

[4] Díaz I, Gascón E, Lázaro S. y Maximiano C. Guía de la Alimentación Mediterránea. Ed. Empresa Pública Desarrollo Agrario y Pesquero. Consejería de Agricultura y Pesca. Junta de Andalucía. 2007.

[5] Hu FB. The Mediterranean diet and mortality–olive oil and beyond. *New Engl J Med.* 2003; 348:2595–96.

[6] Trichopoulou A, Costacou T, Bamia C, Trichopoulou D. Adherence to a Mediterranean diet and survival in a Greek population. *New Engl J Med* 2003; 348:2599–2608.

[7] Trichopoulou A, Naska A, Antoniou A, Friel S, Trygg K y Turrini A. Vegetable and fruit: the evidence in their favour and the public health perspective. *Int J Vitam Nutr Res* 2003; 73:63-9.

[8] Sánchez-Villegas A, Bes-Rastrollo M, Martínez-González MA, Serra-Majem L. Adherence to a Mediterranean dietary pattern and weight gain in a follow-up study: the SUN cohort. *Int J Obe.* 2006; 30:350-8.

[9] Estruch R, Martínez-González MA, Corella D, Salas-Salvadó J, Ruiz-Gutiérrez V, Covas MI, et al. Effects of a Mediterranean-style diet on cardiovascular risk factors: a randomized trial. *Ann Intern Med* 2006; 145:1-11.

[10] Serra-Majem L, Roman B, Estruch R. Scientific evidence of interventions using the Mediterranean diet: a systematic review. *Nutr Rev* 2006; 64:S27-47.

[11] Sofi F, Cesari F, Abbate R, Gensini, GF, Casini A. Adherence to Mediterranean diet and health status: meta-analysis. *BMJ* 2008; 337:a1344

[12] Aranceta J. Spanish food patterns. *Public Health Nutr* 2001;4:1399–1402.

[13] Sánchez-Villegas A, Martinez JA, De Irala I y Martinez-González MA. Determinants of the adherence to an "a priori" defined Mediterranean dietary pattern. *Eur J Nutr.* 2002; 41:249-57.

[14] Tur JA, Serra-Majem L, Romaguera D y Pous A. Does the diet of the Balearic population, a Mediterranean type diet, still provide adequate antioxidant nutrient intakes? *Eur J Nutr* 2005; 44:204-13.

[15] Sofi F, Vecchio S, Giuliani G, Martinelli F, Marcucci R, Gori AM, et al. Dietary habits, lifestyle and cardiovascular risk factors in a clinically healthy Italian population: the "Florence" diet is not Mediterranean. *Eur J Clin Nutr* 2005; 59:584-91.

[16] Bollat P, Durá T. Dietary model of college students. *Nutr Hosp* 2008; 23:619-20.

[17]   Serra-Majem L, García-Closas R, Ribas L, Pérez-Rodrigo C, Aranceta J. Food patterns of Spanish schoolchildren and adolescents: The Enid Study. *Public Health Nutrition* 2001; 4:1433-38.

[18]   Tur JA, Romaguera D y Pons A. Food consumption patterns in a Mediterranean region: does the Mediterranean diet still exist? *Ann Nutr Metab* 2004; 48:193-201.

[19]   Guerra A, Feldl F y Koletzko B. Fatty acid composition of plasma lipids in healthy Portuguese children: is the Mediterranean diet disappearing? *Ann Nutr Metab* 2001; 45:78–81.

[20]   González CA, Argilaga S, Agudo A, Amiano P, Barricarte A, Beguiristain JM, et al. Sociodemographic differences in adherence to the Mediterranean dietary pattern in Spanish populations. *Gac Sanit* 2002; 16:214–21.

[21]   Tur JA, Romaguera D y Pons A. Adherence to the Mediterranean dietary pattern among the population of the Balearic Islands. *Br J Nutr* 2004; 92:341–6.

[22]   Alberti-Fidanza A, Findanza F. Mediterranean Adequacy Index of Italian diets. *Public Health Nutrition* 2004; 7:937–41.

[23]   Gerber M. Qualitative methods to evaluate Mediterranean diet in adults. *Public Health Nutrition* 2006; 9:147–51.

[24]   Bach A, Serra-Majem Ll, Carrasco JL, Roman B, Ngo J, Bertomeu I, et al. The use of indexes evaluating the adherence to the Mediterranean diet in epidemiological studies: a review. *Public Health Nutrition* 2006; 9:132–46.

[25]   Serra-Majem L, Ribas L, Ngo J, Ortega RM, García A, Pérez-Rodrigo C, et al. Food, Youth and the Mediterranean diet in Spain. Development of KIDMED, Mediterranean Diet Quality Index in children and adolescents. *Public Health Nutrition* 2004; 7:931-5.

[26]   Martínez MI, Hernández MD, Ojeda M, Mena R, Alegre A, et al. Development of a program of nutritional education and valuation of the change of healthful nourishing habits in a population of students of Obligatory Secondary Education. *Nutr Hosp* 2009; 24:504-10.

[27]   Serra-Majem LI, Ribas L, García A, Pérez-Rodrigo C, Aranceta J. Nutrient adequacy and Mediterranean Diet in Spanish school children and adolescents. *Eur J Clin Nutr* 2003; 57(Suppl 1):35-9.

[28]   Kontogianni MD, Farmaki AE, Vidra N, Sofrona S, Magkanari F, Yannakoulia M. Associations between lifestyle patterns and body mass index in a sample of Greek children and adolescents. *J Am Diet Assoc* 2010; 110:215-21.

[29] Kontogianni MD, Farmaki AE, Vidra N, Sofrona S, Magkanari F, Yannakoulia M. Associations between lifestyle patterns and body mass index in a sample, Farmaki AE, Koinaki S, Belogianni K, Sofrona S, et al.Adherence rates to the Mediterranean diet are low in a representative sample of Greek children and adolescents. *J Nutr* 2008; 138:1951-56.

[30] 30. Lazarou C, Panagiotakos DB, Matalas AL. Level of adherence to the Mediterranean diet among children from Cyprus: the CYKIDS study. Public *Health Nutr* 2009; 12:991-1000.

[31] Tur JA, Romaguera D, Pons A. The Diet Quality Index-International (DQI-I): is it a useful tool to evaluate the quality of the Mediterranean diet. *Br J Nutr* 2005; 93:369–76.

[32] Ferro-Luzzi A, Branca F. Mediterranean diet, Italian-style: prototype of a healthy. *Am J Clin Nutr* 1995; 61(Suppl):1338-45.

[33] Trichopoulou A. Modified Mediterranean diet and survival: EPIC-elderly prospective cohort study. *BMJ* 2005; 330:991-5.

[34] Sánchez-Villegas A, Delgado-Rodriguez M, Martinez-González MA, De Irala-Estévez J. Gender, age, socio-demographic and lifestyle factors associated with major dietary patterns in the Spanish Project SUN (Seguimiento Universidad de Navarra). *Eur J Nutr* 2003; 57:285-292.

[35] Mariscal-Arcas M, Rivas A, Velasco J, Ortega M, Caballero AM, Olea-Serrano F. Evaluation of the Mediterranean Diet Quality Index (KIDMED) in children and adolescents in Southern Spain. *Public Health Nutrition* 2009; 12:1408–12.

[36] Durá T. Intake of milk and dairy products in a college population. *Nutr Hosp* 2008; 23:91-6.

[37] Ayechu A, Durá T. Mediterranean diet and adolescents. *Nutr Hosp* 2009; 24:759-60.

[38] López J, Gómez P, Castro P, Marín C, Paz E, Bravo MD, et al. Mediterranean diet improves low density lipoprotein susceptibility to oxidative modifications. *Med Clin* (Barc) 2000; 115:361-5.

[39] Nicklas TA, Reger C, Myers y O'Neil C: Breakfast consumption with and without vitamin-mineral supplement use favorably impacts daily nutrient intake of ninth-grade students. *J Adolesc Health* 2000; 27:314-21.

[40] Lazarou C, Panagiotakos DB, Kouta C, Matalas AL. Dietary and other lifestyle characteristics of Cypriot school children: results from the nationwide CYKIDS study. *BMC Public Health.* 2009; 9:147-57.

EDITOR'S CONTACT INFORMATION

Dr. Teodoro Durá-Travé,
School of Medicine, University of Navarra
Department of Pediatrics, Navarra Hospital Complex
Avenue Irunlarrea, 4, Pamplona 31008, Spain
Tel: +34-848-422-563
Fax: +34-848-429-924
Email: tduratra@cfnavarra.es

INDEX

N

S